AGAINST
EMPATHY

AGAINST EMPATHY

The Case for Rational Compassion

PAUL BLOOM

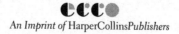
An Imprint of HarperCollinsPublishers

HarperCollins books may be purchased for educational, business, or
sales promotional use. For information please e-mail the Special Markets Department at SPsales@harpercollins.com.

FIRST EDITION

Designed by Joy O'Meara

Library of Congress Cataloging-in-Publication Data has been applied
for.

ISBN 978-0-06-233933-1

17 18 19 20   RRD   10 9 8 7 6 5 4

For my sister,
Elisa Bloom,

who always knows the right thing to do

... empathy is always perched precariously
between gift and invasion.

—Leslie Jamison, *The Empathy Exams*

... human beings are above all reasoning beings ...

—Martha Nussbaum, *Sex and Social Justice*

Contents

AGAINST
EMPATHY

Prologue

I was at home one bright morning a few years ago, avoiding work and surfing the Web, when I heard about the massacre in Newtown, Connecticut. The first reports sounded awful but not unusually so—someone had been shot at a school—but gradually the details came in, and soon I learned that Adam Lanza had killed his mother in her bed at about nine in the morning and then gone to Sandy Hook Elementary School and murdered twenty young children and six adults. Then he killed himself.

There's a lot to be said about what motivated Lanza to do such a horrific thing, but here I am interested in the reactions of the rest of us. My wife wanted to go to our own children's school and take them home. She resisted the urge—our sons were teenagers, and even if they were in elementary school, she knew that this would make no sense. But I understood the impulse. I watched videos of frantic parents running to the crime scene and imagined what that must feel like. Even thinking about it now, my stomach churns. Later that afternoon I was in a coffeehouse near my office, and a woman at a table next to me was sniffling and hoarse, being consoled by a friend, and I heard enough to learn that although she knew nobody at Sandy Hook, she had a child of the same age as those who were murdered.

There will always be events that shock us, such as the terrorist attacks of 9/11 or those many mass shootings that now seem part of everyday life. But for me and the people around me, the murders at Sandy Hook were different. It was an unusually savage crime; it involved children; and it happened close to where we lived. Just about everyone around me had some personal connection to the families of Newtown. We went to a candlelight vigil at the New Haven Green a few days later; my younger son wept, and for months afterward he wore a bracelet in honor of those who died.

I later watched a press conference in which the president choked up as he spoke about the killings, and while I am cynical about politicians, I didn't think for a moment that it was calculated. I was glad to see him so affected.

Our response to that event, at the time and later on, was powerfully influenced by our empathy, by our capacity—many would see it as a gift—to see the world through others' eyes, to feel what they feel. It is easy to see why so many people view empathy as a powerful force for goodness and moral change. It is easy to see why so many believe that the only problem with empathy is that too often we don't have enough of it.

I used to believe this as well. But now I don't. Empathy has its merits. It can be a great source of pleasure, involved in art and fiction and sports, and it can be a valuable aspect of intimate relationships. And it can sometimes spark us to do good. But on the whole, it's a poor moral guide. It grounds foolish judgments and often motivates indifference and cruelty. It can lead to irrational and unfair political decisions, it can corrode certain important relationships, such as between a doctor and a patient, and make us worse at being friends, parents, husbands, and wives. I am against empathy, and one of the goals of this book is to persuade you to be against empathy too.

This is a radical position, but it's not *that* radical. This isn't one of those weird pro-psychopathy books. The argument against empathy isn't that we should be selfish and immoral. It's the opposite. It's that if we want to be good and caring people, if we want to make the world a better place, then we are better off without empathy.

Or to put it more carefully, we are better off without empathy in a certain sense. Some people use *empathy* as referring to everything good, as a synonym for morality and kindness and compassion. And many of the pleas that people make for more empathy just express the view that it would be better if we were nicer to one another. I agree with this!

Others think about empathy as the act of understanding other people, getting inside their heads and figuring out what they are thinking. I'm not against empathy in that sense either. Social intelligence is like any sort of intelligence and can be used as a tool for moral action. We will see, though, that this sort of "cognitive empathy" is overrated as a force for good. After all, the ability to accurately read the desires and motivations of others is a hallmark of the successful psychopath and can be used for cruelty and exploitation.

The notion of empathy that I'm most interested in is the act of feeling what you believe other people feel—experiencing what they experience. This is how most psychologists and philosophers use the term. But I should stress that nothing rests on the word itself. If you'd like to use it in a broader way, to refer to our capacity for caring and love and goodness, or in a narrower way, to refer to the capacity to understand others, well, that's fine. For you, I'm *not* against empathy. You should then think about my arguments as bearing on a psychological process that many people—but not you—think of as empathy. Or you can just forget about terminology altogether and think of this book as a discussion of morality and moral psychology, exploring what it takes to be a good person.

The idea I'll explore is that the act of feeling what you think others are feeling—whatever one chooses to call this—is different from being compassionate, from being kind, and most of all, from being good. From a moral standpoint, we're better off without it.

Many people see this as an unlikely claim. Empathy in this sense is a capacity that many believe to be vitally important. It is often said that the rich don't make the effort to appreciate what it is like to be poor, and if they did we would have more equality and social justice. When there are shootings of unarmed black men, commentators on the left argue that the police don't have enough empathy for black teenagers, while those on the right argue that the critics of the police don't have enough empathy for what it's like to work as a police officer, having to face difficult and stressful and dangerous situations. It's said that whites don't have enough empathy for blacks and that men don't have enough empathy for women. Many commentators would agree with Barack Obama that the clash between Israelis and Palestinians will only end when those on each side "learn to stand in each other's shoes." In a few chapters, we'll meet a psychologist who argues that if only the Nazis had had more empathy, the Holocaust would never have happened. There are many who maintain that if doctors and therapists had more empathy, they would be better at their jobs, and if certain politicians had more empathy, they wouldn't be endorsing such rotten policies. Certainly many of us feel that if the people in our lives had more empathy for our situations—if they could really feel what our lives are like—they would treat us a lot better.

I think this is all mistaken. The problems we face as a society and as individuals are rarely due to lack of empathy. Actually, they are often due to too much of it.

This isn't just an attack on empathy. There is a broader agenda here. I want to make a case for the value of conscious, deliberative reasoning in everyday life, arguing that we should strive to use our heads rather than our hearts. We do this a lot already, but we should work on doing more.

This is an unfashionable position; some would call it ignorant and naive. Many of my colleagues argue that our most important judgments and actions emerge from neural processes that are not accessible to our conscious selves. Sigmund Freud gets credit for advancing the strong version of this claim, but it's been resurrected in modern times, sometimes in the most extreme forms. I've lost count of how many times I've heard some philosopher, critic, or public intellectual state that psychologists have proved we are not rational beings.

This rejection of reason is particularly strong in the moral domain. It is now accepted by many that our judgments of right and wrong are determined by gut feelings of empathy, anger, disgust, and love, and that deliberation and rationality are largely irrelevant. As Frans de Waal puts it, we don't live in an age of reason, we live in an age of empathy.

It might feel, at least to some of us, that our opinions about issues such as abortion and the death penalty are the product of careful deliberation and that our specific moral acts, such as deciding to give to charity or visit a friend in the hospital—or for that matter, deciding to shoplift or shout a racist insult out of a car window—are grounded in conscious decision-making. But this is said to be mistaken. As Jonathan Haidt argues, we are not judges; we are lawyers, making up explanations after the deeds have been done. Reason is impotent. "We celebrate rationality," agrees de Waal, "but when push comes to shove we assign it little weight."

Some scholars will go on to reassure us that the emotional nature of morality is a good thing. Morality is the sort of thing that one shouldn't think through. Many of our moral heroes, real and fictional, are not rational maximizers or ethical egg-heads; they are people of heart. From Huckleberry Finn to Pip to Jack Bauer, from Jesus to Gandhi to Martin Luther King Jr., they are individuals of great feeling. Rationality gets you Hanni-bal Lecter and Lex Luther.

Now, I don't think this perspective on mind and morality is entirely wrong. Much of moral judgment is not the result of conscious deliberation. In fact, my last book, *Just Babies*, was about the origin of moral understanding, and I argued there that even babies have some sense of right and wrong—and babies don't do conscious deliberation. There is a lot of evidence that the foundations of morality have evolved through the process of natural selection. We didn't think them up.

It's clear as well that emotions play a powerful role in our moral lives—and that sometimes this is a good thing. The necessity of feeling has been defended by Confucius and other Chinese scholars of his period and by the philosophers of the Scottish Enlightenment, and it has been further supported by contemporary work in cognitive science and neuroscience. There are many demonstrations, for instance, that damage to parts of the brain involving the emotions can have a devastating effect on people's lives. There are also recent studies by my colleague David Rand that find that our instinctive gut decision is often a kind and cooperative one; slow deliberation sometimes makes us act worse.

But I wrote the book you are holding because I believe our emotional nature has been oversold. We have gut feelings, but we also have the capacity to override them, to think through issues, including moral issues, and to come to conclusions that can surprise us. I think this is where the real action is. It's what makes us distinctively human, and it gives us the potential to be better to one another, to create a world with less suffering and more flourishing and happiness.

There is nothing more natural, for instance, than the priority we give to our friends and family. Nobody could doubt that we care about those close to us much more than we care about strangers. The influence of kinship is expressed in the phrase "Blood is thicker than water," while the pull of reciprocity was nicely summarized in a toast that I learned as a child from one of my favorite relatives:

Here's to those who wish us well.
All the rest can go to hell.

From a Darwinian perspective, these preferences are no-brainers. Creatures who favor their own are at a huge advantage over those who are impartial. If there ever arose a human who was indifferent to friend versus stranger, to his child versus another child, his genes got trounced by the genes of those who cared more for their own. This is why we are not natural-born egalitarians.

These parochial desires don't ever go away, and perhaps never should go away. We'll get to this later, but I'm not sure what one should think about a person who doesn't have any special love for friends and family, who cares for everyone equally. Some would see such a person as a saint. Others, including myself, think this goes too far, and there's something almost repellent about living one's life that way.

But regardless, these innate preferences don't define us. We are smart enough to intellectually grasp that the lives of those in faraway lands (people who aren't related to us, don't know us, don't wish us well) matter just as much as the lives of our children. They really shouldn't go to hell. We can appreciate that favoring one's own ethnic group or race, however natural and intuitive it feels, can be unfair and immoral. And we can act to enforce impartiality—for instance, by creating policies that establish certain principles of impartial justice.

We are emotional creatures, then, but we are also rational beings, with the capacity for rational decision-making. We can override, deflect, and overrule our passions, and we often should do so. It's not hard to see this for feelings like anger and hate—it's clear that these can lead us astray, that we do better when they don't rule us and when we are capable of circumventing them. But it would really nail down the case in favor of rationality to show that it's true as well for something as seemingly positive as empathy. That is one of the reasons I have written this book.

I am going to argue three things, then. First, our moral decisions and actions are powerfully shaped by the force of empathy. Second, this often makes the world worse. And, third, we have the capacity to do better.

But how could empathy steer us wrong? Well, read on. But in brief: Empathy is a spotlight focusing on certain people in the here and now. This makes us care more about them, but it leaves us insensitive to the long-term consequences of our acts and blind as well to the suffering of those we do not or cannot empathize with. Empathy is biased, pushing us in the direction of parochialism and racism. It is shortsighted, motivating actions that might make things better in the short term but lead to tragic results in the future. It is innumerate, favoring the one over the many. It can spark violence; our empathy for those close to us is a powerful force for war and atrocity toward others. It is corrosive in personal relationships; it exhausts the spirit and can diminish the force of kindness and love.

When you're done with this book, you might ask what's *not* wrong with empathy.

Now we will never live in a world without empathy—or without anger, shame, or hate for that matter. And I wouldn't want to live in such a world. All these sentiments add to our lives in various ways. But I do think we can create a culture where these emotions are put in their proper place, and this book is a step in that direction.

I said that this view is unfashionable, but I'm hardly a lone voice in the wilderness, and I'm far from the first to pursue this sort of critique. There are many who have made the case for the unreliability of empathy, such as Richard Davidson, Sam Harris, Jesse Prinz, and Peter Singer, and those who have argued for the centrality of reason in everyday life, such as Michael Lynch and Michael Shermer. It's reassuring to have these scholars on my side. Others have done the work of outlining empathy's limits and of carefully distinguishing empathy from other capacities, such as compassion and a sense of justice. I'm thinking here of Jean Decety, David DeSteno, Joshua Greene, Martin Hoffman, Larissa MacFarquhar, Martha Nussbaum, and Steven Pinker. I am particularly impressed by the research of Tania Singer, a cognitive neuroscientist, and Matthieu Ricard, a Buddhist monk—two scholars working together to explore the distinction between empathy and compassion. I've been influenced as well by a novelist, Leslie Jamison, and a literary scholar, Elaine Scarry, both of whom have fascinating things to say about empathy and its limits.

This book contains six chapters and two interludes. Of course, you should read them all. But in a pinch, they can be treated as independent essays.

The first lays out the attack on empathy in broad strokes—if you read one chapter, this should be it. The second and third zoom in, presenting the psychology and neuroscience of empathy and exploring the features that make it inadequate as a moral guide. This is followed by a short interlude exploring the relationship between empathy and politics, addressing the view that liberals are more empathic than conservatives.

The fourth chapter is about empathy and intimacy. This is followed by another interlude on a topic that I can't seem to get away from—the moral lives of babies and children.

The fifth chapter is about evil, looking skeptically at the view that lack of empathy makes people worse.

The final chapter steps back to defend human rationality, arguing that we really do have the capacity to use reasoned deliberation to make it through the world. We live in an age of reason.

One of the many pleasures of writing a book like this is that it takes one in surprising directions. In the pages that follow you'll find discussions about the roots of war, the relationship between apologies and sadism, what neuroscience has to say about decision-making, the moral psychology of Buddhism, and much else. Who says a book has to be about just one thing?

More than anything else I've written, what you see here is the product of conversation and criticism. For a year before I started to write it, and then in the course of the writing, I've published articles in popular outlets describing earlier versions of these ideas—in *The New Yorker* (looking at policy issues), the *Boston Review* (looking at intimate relations), *The Atlantic* (defending the role of reason, exploring how empathy can motivate violence), and the *New York Times* (on the problems we have understanding the mental states of others). Some parts of these articles have found their way here, though all of them have been modified, sometimes substantially so, as the result of the responses I received and the conversations I got into.

One thing I learned from the reactions to these earlier articles is that many people think my attack on empathy is ridiculous. When my *New Yorker* article went online, I checked out Twitter to see the reaction, and the first comment that linked to the article said: "Possibly the dumbest thing I ever read." In response to the *Boston Review* article, one sociologist blogger called me "an intellectual disgrace and moral monster." I've been described as an apologist for psychopathy and predatory capitalism, and people have made unkind speculations about my childhood and personal life.

Some of the counterarguments, even those by the nastiest people, turned out to be good ones. (As Fredrik deBoer once put it, "Your haters are your closest readers.") I have changed my mind about some of my earlier positions, and even when I wasn't convinced, the criticisms helped me understand what people tend to object to. I'm sure there will be new objections, but I try here to anticipate, and respond to, at least some of the concerns that will occur to a thoughtful reader.

The most common critical response, which I've received from critics, friends, and students, is that I've gone too far. Perhaps I've shown that empathy, characterized in a certain way, might lead us astray. But nothing is perfect. Maybe the problem is that we sometimes rely on empathy too much, or that we sometimes use it in the wrong way. What one should do, then, is put it in its proper place. Not *Against Empathy* but *Against the Misapplication of Empathy*. Or *Empathy Is Not Everything*. Or *Empathy Plus Reason Make a Great Combination*. Empathy is like cholesterol, with a good type and a bad type.

I'm somewhat swayed by this. I will occasionally discuss some positive aspects of empathy. There are situations where people's empathy can motivate good action, and moral individuals can use empathy as a tool to motivate others to do the right thing. Empathy might play a valuable, perhaps irreplaceable, role in intimate relationships. And empathy can be a source of great pleasure. It's not all bad.

But still, I stand fast. On balance, empathy is a negative in human affairs. It's not cholesterol. It's sugary soda, tempting and delicious and bad for us. Now I'll tell you why.

CHAPTER 1

Other People's Shoes

For the last couple of years, when people ask me what I've been up to, I say that I'm writing a book. They ask for details and I tell them, "It's about empathy." They tend to smile and nod when I say the word, and then I add: "I'm against it."

This usually gets a laugh. I was surprised at this response at first, but I've learned that being against empathy is like being against kittens—a view considered so outlandish that it can't be serious. It's certainly a position that's easy to misunderstand. So I'll be clear from the start: I am not against morality, compassion, kindness, love, being a good neighbor, being a mensch, and doing the right thing. Actually, I'm writing this book because I'm for all those things. I want to make the world a better place. I've just come to believe that relying on empathy is the wrong way to do it.

One reason why being against empathy is so shocking is that people often assume that empathy is an absolute good. You can never be too rich or too thin . . . or too empathic.

Empathy is unusual in this regard. We are more critical when it comes to judging other feelings, emotions, and capacities. We recognize their nuances. Anger can drive a father to beat his infant son to death, but anger at injustice can transform the world. Admiration can be wonderful if directed toward someone who deserves it; less wonderful if one is admiring, say, a serial killer. I am a fan of deliberative reasoning and will push for its importance throughout the book, but I'll admit that it too can steer us wrong. Robert Jay Lifton, in *The Nazi Doctors*, talks about the struggles of those who performed experiments on prisoners in concentration camps. He describes these doctors as smart people who used their intelligence to talk themselves into doing terrible things. They would have been better off listening to their hearts.

For just about any human capacity, you can assess the pros and cons. So let's give empathy the same scrutiny.

To do so, we have to be clear what we mean by *empathy*. There are many definitions thought up by psychologists and philosophers: One book on the topic lists nine different meanings of the word. One team of researchers notes that *empathy* is used for everything "from yawning contagion in dogs, to distress signaling in chickens, to patient-centered attitudes in human medicine." Another team notes that "there are probably nearly as many definitions of empathy as people working on this topic." But the differences are often subtle, and the sense of empathy that I'll be talking about throughout this book is the most typical one. Empathy is *the act of coming to experience the world as you think someone else does*.

Empathy in this sense was explored in detail by the philosophers of the Scottish Enlightenment, though they called it "sympathy." As Adam Smith put it, we have the capacity to think about another person and "place ourselves in his situation . . .

and become in some measure the same person with him, and thence form some idea of his sensations, and even feel something which, though weaker in degree, is not altogether unlike them."

That is how I'm thinking about empathy. But there is a related sense that has to do with the capacity to appreciate what's going on in the minds of other people without any contagion of feeling. If your suffering makes me suffer, if I feel what you feel, that's empathy in the sense that I'm interested in here. But if I understand that you are in pain without feeling it myself, this is what psychologists describe as social cognition, social intelligence, mind reading, theory of mind, or mentalizing. It's also sometimes described as a form of empathy—"cognitive empathy" as opposed to "emotional empathy," which is most of my focus.

Later in this chapter, I'll talk about cognitive empathy, rather critically, but right now we should just keep in mind that these two sorts of empathy are distinct—they emerge from different brain processes, they influence us in different ways, and you can have a lot of one and a little of the other.

Empathy—in the Adam Smith sense, the "emotional empathy" sense—can occur automatically, even involuntarily. Smith describes how "persons of delicate fibres" who notice a beggar's sores and ulcers "are apt to feel an itching or uneasy sensation in the correspondent part of their own bodies." John Updike writes, "My grandmother would have choking fits at the kitchen table, and my own throat would feel narrow in sympathy." When Nicholas Epley goes to his children's soccer games, he has to leave the row in front of him clear for "empathy kicks." And it takes someone sturdier than me to watch someone bash himself on the thumb with a hammer without flinching.

But empathy is more than a reflex. It can be nurtured, stanched, developed, and extended through the imagination. It can be focused and directed by acts of will. In a speech before he became president, Barack Obama described how empathy can be a choice. He stressed how important it is "to see the world through the eyes of those who are different from us—the child who's hungry, the steelworker who's been laid off, the family who lost the entire life they built together when the storm came to town. When you think like this—when you choose to broaden your ambit of concern and empathize with the plight of others, whether they are close friends or distant strangers—it becomes harder not to act, harder not to help."

I like this quote because it provides a nice illustration of how empathy can be a force for good. Empathy makes us care more about other people, more likely to try to improve their lives.

A few years ago, Steven Pinker began a discussion of empathy with a list:

> Here is a sample of titles and subtitles that have appeared in just the past two years: The Age of Empathy, Why Empathy Matters, The Social Neuroscience of Empathy, The Science of Empathy, The Empathy Gap, Why Empathy Is Essential (and Endangered), Empathy in the Global World, and How Companies Prosper When They Create Widespread Empathy. . . . [Other examples include] Teaching Empathy, Teaching Children Empathy, and The Roots of Empathy: Changing the World Child by Child, whose author, according to an endorsement by the pediatrician T.

Berry Brazelton, "strives to bring about no less than world peace and protection for our planet's future, starting with schools and classrooms everywhere, one child, one parent, one teacher at a time."

As I started to write this book, I kept my eyes out for similar examples. Right now, there are over fifteen hundred books on amazon.com with *empathy* in their title or subtitle. Looking at the top twenty, there are books for parents and teachers, self-help guides, marketing books ("How to use empathy to create products people love"), and even a couple of good scientific books.

There are many Web pages, blogs, and YouTube channels devoted to championing empathy, such as a website that lists everything Barack Obama has said about empathy, including this famous quote: "The biggest deficit that we have in our society and in the world right now is an empathy deficit." After I published an article that explored some of the ideas in this book, I was invited to join a series of "empathy circles": online conversations in which individuals talk about the importance of empathy and work self-consciously to be empathic toward each other. Books on empathy fill my shelves and my iPad, and I've been to several conferences with "Empathy" in their names.

I became sensitive to the way empathy is discussed in response to certain public events. In the fall of 2014, there was a series of incidents in which unarmed black men died at the hands of the police, and many people expressed their anguish about the lack of empathy that Americans—and particularly police officers—have with racial minorities. But I would read as well angry responses complaining about the lack of empathy that many Americans have with the police, or with the victims of crimes. The one thing everyone could agree on, it seemed, was that more empathy is needed.

Many believe that empathy will save the world, and this is particularly the case for those who champion liberal or progressive causes. Giving advice to liberal politicians, George Lakoff writes, "Behind every progressive policy lies a single moral value: empathy. . . ." Jeremy Rifkin calls for us to make the "leap to global empathic consciousness," and he ends his book *The Empathic Civilization* with the plaintive question "Can we reach biosphere consciousness and global empathy in time to avoid global collapse?"

For every specific problem, lack of empathy is seen as the diagnosis and more empathy as the cure. Emily Bazelon writes "The scariest aspect of bullying is the total lack of empathy" — a diagnosis she applies not only to the bullies but to those who do nothing to help the victims. The solution, she suggests, is "to remember that almost everyone has the capacity for empathy and decency — and to tend that seed as best as we possibly can." Andrew Solomon explores the trials of children who are different in critical ways from their parents (such as dwarfs, transgender children, and children with Down syndrome). He worries that we live in xenophobic times and diagnoses "a crisis of empathy." But he suggests as well that these special children can help address the empathy crisis and notes that parents of such children report an increase in empathy and compassion. This argument is familiar to me: My brother is severely autistic, and when I was growing up I heard it said that such children are a blessing from God — they teach us to be empathic to those who are different from us.

Perhaps the most extreme claim about lack of empathy is

advanced by Simon Baron-Cohen. For him, evil individuals are nothing more than people who lack empathy. His answer to the question "What is evil?" is "empathy erosion."

It makes sense that empathy would be seen by so many as the magic bullet of morality. The argument in its simplest form goes like this: Everyone is naturally interested in him- or herself; we care most about our own pleasure and pain. It requires nothing special to yank one's hand away from a flame or to reach for a glass of water when thirsty. But empathy makes the experiences of others salient and important—your pain becomes my pain, your thirst becomes my thirst, and so I rescue you from the fire or give you something to drink. Empathy guides us to treat others as we treat ourselves and hence expands our selfish concerns to encompass other people.

In this way, the willful exercise of empathy can motivate kindness that would never have otherwise occurred. Empathy can make us care about a slave, or a homeless person, or someone in solitary confinement. It can put us into the mind of a gay teenager bullied by his peers, or a victim of rape. We can empathize with a member of a despised minority or someone suffering from religious persecution in a faraway land. All these experiences are alien to me, but through the exercise of empathy, I can, in some limited way, experience them myself, and this makes me a better person. In *Leaves of Grass*, Walt Whitman put it like this: "I do not ask the wounded person how he feels. I myself become the wounded person."

Empathy can be used to motivate others to do good. Just about all parents have at some point reminded children of the consequences of bad acts, prodding them with remarks like "How would you feel if someone did that to you?" Martin Hoffman estimates that these empathic prompts occur about four thousand times a year in the average child's life. Every charity, every political movement, every social cause will use empathy to motivate action.

And there's more! I haven't yet told you about the laboratory research, the cognitive neuroscience studies, the philosophical analyses, the research with babies and chimps and rats—all said to demonstrate the importance of empathy in making us good.

Even the biggest fan of empathy should admit that there are other possible motivations for good action. To use a classic example from philosophy—first thought up by the Chinese philosopher Mencius—imagine that you are walking by a lake and see a young child struggling in shallow water. If you can easily wade into the water and save her, you should do it. It would be wrong to keep walking.

What motivates this good act? It is possible, I suppose, that you might imagine what it feels like to be drowning, or anticipate what it would be like to be the child's mother or father hearing that she drowned. Such empathic feelings could then motivate you to act. But that is hardly necessary. You don't need empathy to realize that it's wrong to let a child drown. Any normal person would just wade in and scoop up the child, without bothering with any of this empathic hoo-ha.

More generally, as Jesse Prinz and others have pointed out, we are capable of all sorts of moral judgments that aren't grounded in empathy. Many wrongs, after all, have no distinct victims to empathize with. We disapprove of people who shoplift or cheat on their taxes, throw garbage out of their car windows, or jump ahead in line—even if there is no specific person who apprecia-bly suffers because of their actions, nobody to empathize with.

And so there has to be more to morality than empathy. Our decisions about what's right and what's wrong, and our motiva-tions to act, have many sources. One's morality can be rooted in a religious worldview or a philosophical one. It can be motivated by a more diffuse concern for the fates of others—something of-ten described as concern or compassion and which I will argue is a better moral guide than empathy.

To see this at work, consider that there are people who are acting right now to make the world better in the future, who worry that we are making the planet hotter or running out of fos-sil fuels or despoiling the environment or failing to respond to the rise of extreme religious groups. These worries have nothing to do with an empathic connection with anyone in particular—because there is no particular person to feel empathic toward—but are instead rooted in a more general concern about human lives and human flourishing.

In some cases, empathy-based concerns clash with other sorts of moral concerns. As I write this, there is a debate going around in the academic community over whether professors should an-nounce in advance that material presented in the lecture hall or seminar room might be upsetting to certain people, particu-larly those with a history of trauma, so that the students have a chance to absent themselves from class during that period.

The arguments in favor of these "trigger warnings" have largely been based on empathy. Imagine what it would be like to be the victim of rape and suddenly your professor—in a class that isn't about rape at all—shows a movie clip depicting a sex-ual assault. It might be terrible. And you would have to either sit through it or go through the humiliating experience of walking out in the middle of the class. If you feel empathy for a student in this situation, as I imagine any normal person would, this would make you receptive to the idea that trigger warnings are a good idea.

One scholar derisively summed up the move toward trigger warnings as "'empathetic correctness.'" She argues that "instead of challenging the status quo by demanding texts that question the comfort of the Western canon, students are . . . refusing to read texts that challenge their own personal comfort." But this is too dismissive. While concerns about "personal comfort" might be poor reasons to restructure the curriculum, real suffering and anguish are a different story and certainly have to have some weight.

What about the arguments against trigger warnings? These are also about the welfare of people—what else could they be, ultimately?—but they aren't inherently empathic, as they don't connect to concerns about any individual person. Instead, they rest on considerations that are long term, procedural, and abstract. Critics claim that trigger warnings violate the spirit of academia, in which students benefit from being challenged by new experiences. They worry that since it's impossible to anticipate what will set people off, they are impractical. They argue that by focusing on trigger warnings, colleges and universities will divert attention from more important issues, such as better mental health care for students.

Of course, someone making such arguments can try to evoke empathy for individuals, real or imagined—in moral debate, empathy is a spice that makes anything taste better. But concern for specific individuals is not, ultimately, what the anti-trigger-warning arguments are about, so this debate illustrates that there is more than one way to motivate moral concern.

As another example of how empathy can clash with other moral considerations, C. Daniel Batson and his colleagues did an experiment in which they told subjects about a ten-year-old girl named Sheri Summers who had a fatal disease and was waiting in line for treatment that would relieve her pain. Subjects were told that they could move her to the front of the line. When simply asked what to do, they acknowledged that she had to wait because other more needy children were ahead of her. But if they were first asked to imagine what she felt, they tended to choose to move her up, putting her ahead of children who were presumably more deserving. Here empathy was more powerful than fairness, leading to a decision that most of us would see as immoral.

There are all sorts of real-world acts of kindness that are not prompted by empathic concern. We sometimes miss these cases because we are too quick to credit an action to empathy when actually something else is going on. Leslie Jamison, author of *The Empathy Exams*, describes going to a talk by Jason Baldwin, a man who was falsely imprisoned for many years: "I stood up to tell him how much I admired his capacity for forgiveness—I was thinking of his seemingly intuitive ability to forgive the people who'd assumed his guilt—and I asked him where that forgiveness had come from. I was thinking about the stuff I'm always thinking about: webs of empathy, forays of imagination, all the systems by which we inhabit the minds of others. But Baldwin said something quite different, and much simpler: his faith in Christ."

Or consider Zell Kravinsky, who gave almost all of his forty-five-million-dollar fortune to charity. Frustrated that he wasn't doing enough, he then arranged to donate one of his kidneys to a stranger, over the strenuous objections of his family. It's tempting to see someone like this as a super-empath, deeply moved by his feelings about other people. But at least in the case of Kravinsky, it's the opposite. Peter Singer describes him like this: "Kravinsky is a brilliant man: he has one doctorate in education and another on the poetry of John Milton. . . . [H]e puts his altruism in mathematical terms. Quoting scientific studies that show the risk of dying as a result of making a kidney donation to be only 1 in 4,000, he says that not making the donation would have meant he valued his life at 4,000 times that of a stranger, a valuation he finds totally unjustified."

Singer goes further and argues that individuals like Kravinsky, motivated by their cold logic and reasoning, actually do more to help people than those who are gripped by empathic feelings—a proposal that we will return to over and over again throughout this book.

And so there is more to kindness and morality than empathy. To think otherwise is either to define empathy so broadly as to gut it of all content or to have a parched and unimaginative view of the moral psyche. We are complex beings, and there are many routes to moral judgment and moral action.

But a reasonable response at this point might be to concede that while empathy isn't all there is to morality, it is the most important thing. When faced with empathy versus religion or empathy versus reason or empathy versus more distanced compassion, then either there will be no conflict at all or, if there is a conflict, then empathy should win. You might think, for instance, that in the trigger-warning debate I described, the empathy side just has to be the right one. And you might question the morality of someone who helps others but does so without the push of empathy. Some would sneer at Baldwin for being motivated by religious belief, while others would wonder whether Kravinsky, who is almost a caricature of the bloodless utilitarian, maximizing the utility of strangers at the expense of his wife and children, is such a good guy after all.

So how can we put empathy to the test? One way is to look at its consequences. If empathy makes the world a better place, then its defenders are vindicated. But if it turns out that the exercise of empathy makes the world worse, that it leads to more suffering and less thriving, more pain and less happiness, this would be a good reason to seek out alternatives.

When it comes to morality, after all, nobody can doubt that consequences matter. If someone were to wonder why you should save the drowning child—the sort of question only a philosopher would ask, I suppose—one good answer is that if you let her die, things would be worse. She would have lost out on all the good things that come from being alive, and there would be terrible suffering on the part of others. By wading in and pulling her out, you avert all those awful consequences.

Often the consequences of our actions are uncertain. As Yogi Berra once put it: "It's tough to make predictions, especially about the future." A young man has serious problems with drugs and gets arrested; his wealthy parents bail him out. Or they don't; they leave him in prison overnight so that he learns a lesson. A woman decides to have an abortion; a student cheats on an exam that he needs to pass to keep his scholarship; a man leaves Wall Street to join the seminary. The consequences of such actions are hard to anticipate, so it's often hard to know what's right.

In other cases, one can be pretty confident about consequences, so some decisions are easy. Other things being equal, it's better to save one hundred lives than just one; it's wrong to rape, drive drunk, or set people's houses on fire. But there will always be some uncertainty, and when we try to do good, we are like poker players in our aspiration to choose wisely in the face of factors out of our control. In Texas hold 'em, a pair of aces is the best possible starting hand, so if you are holding American Airlines and someone goes all in, you should surely call—but you will sometimes lose because you can't predict what other cards will turn up, and actually, even against a random hand, aces will lose 15 percent of the time. Even if you lose, though, calling was the right choice. The bad outcome just means that you were unlucky.

Similarly, if you save the drowning girl and she grows up to be a genocidal dictator and destroys the world, that's an unlucky outcome, what poker players call "a bad beat," but still, the choice was a good one. When I first thought of this drowning-baby-becomes-dictator example, it was meant as the sort of goofy hypothetical that gets brought up in philosophical seminars, but a graduate student pointed me to an article describing how in Passau, Germany, in the winter of 1894, a four-year-old child playing tag fell through the ice of a frozen river and was rescued by a local priest named Johann Kuehberger—"a brave comrade" as a local paper described him. According to some sources, the child was Adolf Hitler.

In general, then, one way to try to be good and do good is to attend to the consequences of one's actions. This way of thinking about right and wrong is sometimes called "consequentialism," and it has been defended in various forms by Jeremy Bentham, John Stuart Mill, and Henry Sidgwick, and more recently by contemporary philosophers such as Peter Singer and Shelly Kagan. These philosophers disagree about critical details, but they share the view that maximizing good results, fundamentally, is what morality is all about.

Now, not everyone is a consequentialist. Some people adopt the view that we should think about how to act in terms of certain principles, without reference to consequences. Immanuel Kant famously argued, for instance, that lying is wrong regardless of the results. Some would say the same about torture — regardless of what sort of ticking bomb scenario one might think of, regardless of how many lives one might save by sticking needles under the fingernails of some prisoner, still, torture is wrong, and we should never do it.

Certainly our everyday sense of whether an act is right or wrong has to do with more than consequences. There is an obvious moral difference between killing someone on purpose and killing someone through an unavoidable accident (you lose control of your car on an icy road), even though the person is just as dead either way. And there are many cases where the logic of consequentialism leads to answers that clash with heartfelt moral intuitions. We'll discuss some of these, having to do with our felt obligations to friends and family, later on.

There's a lot to be said about these issues, but I'll just note two things here. First, the gap between consequentialism and principle-based moral views might not be as large as it first seems. Many seemingly nonconsequentialist abstract principles can actually be defended in consequentialist terms; they can be seen as useful rules that we are better off applying absolutely, even if they sometimes make things worse. Think about a rule like "Always stop at a red light." In a sense this isn't very consequentialist; when the road is clear and you need to get home on time, it's best overall if you just keep driving. But still, it makes good sense for a society to enforce an absolute rule rather than trusting people to figure it for themselves. The benefits of people not making foolish mistakes outweigh the costs of some lost time at intersections. Maybe we should think about "do not torture" in the same way: Even if there are cases in which torture would be justified, we are all better off with an absolute prohibition.

Second, regardless of what abstract moral principles there are, nobody denies that consequences *also* matter. If Immanuel Kant had to decide whether to hurt someone mildly or kill her, he might well complain that both acts are wrong, but I assume that he would agree that the second is worse. (If not, so much the worst for Kant.)

So what *are* the consequences of empathy? Does it make the world a better place?

It certainly looks like it. After all, empathy drives people to treat others' suffering as if it were their own, which then motivates action to make the suffering go away. I see the bullied teenager and might be tempted initially to join in with his tormenters, out of sadism or boredom or a desire to dominate or be popular, but then I empathize—I feel his pain, I feel what it's like to be bullied—so I don't add to his suffering. Maybe I even rise to his defense. Empathy is like a spotlight directing attention and aid to where it's needed.

But spotlights have a narrow focus, and this is one problem with empathy. It does poorly in a world where there are many people in need and where the effects of one's actions are diffuse, often delayed, and difficult to compute, a world in which an act that helps one person in the here and now can lead to greater suffering in the future.

Further, spotlights only illuminate what they are pointed at, so empathy reflects our biases. Although we might intellectually believe that the suffering of our neighbor is just as awful as the suffering of someone living in another country, it's far easier to empathize with those who are close to us, those who are similar to us, and those we see as more attractive or vulnerable and less scary. Intellectually, a white American might believe that a black person matters just as much as a white person, but he or she will typically find it a lot easier to empathize with the plight of the latter than the former. In this regard, empathy distorts our moral judgments in pretty much the same way that prejudice does.

Empathy is limited as well in that it focuses on specific individuals. Its spotlight nature renders it innumerate and myopic: It doesn't resonate properly to the effects of our actions on groups of people, and it is insensitive to statistical data and estimated costs and benefits.

To see these weaknesses, consider the example that I raised in the prologue, the murders of twenty children and six adults at Sandy Hook Elementary School in Newtown, Connecticut, in 2012. Why did this give rise to such a powerful reaction? It was a mass shooting, and over the last thirty years in the United

States, these have caused hundreds of deaths. This is horrible, but the toll from these mass shootings equals about one-tenth of 1 percent of American homicides, a statistical nonevent. (That is, if you could wave a magic wand and end all mass shootings forever, nobody looking at the overall homicide rates would even notice.) Actually, in the year of the Sandy Hook killings, more schoolchildren were murdered in one American city — Chicago — than were murdered in Newtown, and yet I've never thought about those murdered Chicago children before looking that up, and I'm not likely to think about them again . . . while my mind often drifts back to Newtown. Why?

Part of the answer is that Sandy Hook was a single event. The murders in Chicago are more of a steady background noise. We're constituted so that novel and unusual events catch our attention and trigger our emotional responses.

But it's also in large part because it's easy for people like me to empathize with the children and teachers and parents of Newtown: They're so much like those I know and love. Teenage black kids in Chicago, not so much.

What people did in response to the Newtown massacre also reflects the limitations of empathy. The town was inundated with so much charity that it added to their burden. Hundreds of volunteers had to be recruited to store the gifts and toys that got sent to the city, which kept arriving despite pleas from Newtown officials for people to stop. A vast warehouse was crammed with plush toys that the townspeople had no use for; millions of dollars rolled in to this relatively affluent community. There was a dark comedy here, with people from far poorer communities sending their money to much richer people, guided by the persistent itch of empathic concern.

Now one reasonable reaction to this is that empathy isn't to blame for this sort of irrational and disproportionate response. The real problem is that we don't have enough empathy for other people. We should empathize with the children and families of Newtown, but we should *also* empathize with the children and families in Chicago. While we're at it, we should empathize with billions of other people around the world, in Bangladesh and Pyongyang and the Sudan. We should empathize with the elderly who don't get enough food, the victims of religious persecution, the poor without adequate health care, the rich who suffer from existential angst, the victims of sexual assault, those falsely accursed of sexual assault . . .

But we can't. Intellectually, we can value the lives of all these individuals; we can give them weight when we make decisions. But what we can't do is empathize with all of them. Indeed, you cannot empathize with more than one or two people at the same time. Try it. Think about someone you know who's going through a difficult time and try to feel what she or he is feeling. Feel that person's pain. Now at the same time do this with someone else who's in a difficult situation, with different feelings and experiences. Can you simultaneously empathize with two people? If so, good, congratulations. Now add a third person to the mix. Now try ten. And then a hundred, a thousand, a million. Several years ago, Annie Dillard mocked the very idea: "There are 1,198,500,000 people alive now in China. To get a feel for what this means, simply take yourself—in all your singularity, importance, complexity, and love—and multiply by 1,198,500,000. See? Nothing to it."

If God exists, maybe He can simultaneously feel the pain and pleasure of every sentient being. But for us mortals, empathy really is a spotlight. It's a spotlight that has a narrow focus, one that shines most brightly on those we love and gets dim for those who are strange or different or frightening.

It would be bad enough if empathy were simply silent when faced with problems involving large numbers, but actually it's worse. It can sway us toward the one over the many. This perverse moral mathematics is part of the reason why governments and individuals care more about a little girl stuck in a well than about events that will affect millions or billions. It is why outrage at the suffering of a few individuals can lead to actions, such as going to war, that have terrible consequences for many more.

Empathy is particularly insensitive to consequences that apply statistically rather than to specific individuals. Imagine learning that a faulty vaccine has caused Rebecca Smith, an adorable eight-year-old, to get extremely sick. If you watch her suffering and listen to her and her family, the empathy will flow, and you'll want to act. But suppose that stopping the vaccine program will cause, say, a dozen random children to die. Here your empathy is silent—how can you empathize with a statistical abstraction? To the extent that you can appreciate that it's better for one specific child to die than for an unknown and imprecise larger number of children to die, you are using capacities other than empathy.

Or consider Willie Horton. In 1987 Horton, a convicted murderer, was released on furlough from the Northeastern Correctional Center in Massachusetts and raped a woman after attacking and tying up her fiancé. The furlough program came to be seen as a humiliating mistake on the part of Governor Michael Dukakis and was used against him by his opponents during his subsequent run for president.

Yet the program may have reduced the likelihood of such incidents. A report at the time found that the recidivism rate in Massachusetts had dropped in the fifteen years after the program was introduced and that convicts who were furloughed before being released were less likely to go on to commit a crime than those who were not. On balance, then, the world was better—fewer murders and fewer rapes—when the program was in place. But we react empathically to the victims of Horton's actions, while our empathy is silent when it comes to the individuals who weren't raped, assaulted, or killed as a result of the program.

The issues here go beyond policy. I'll argue that what really matters for kindness in our everyday interactions is not empathy but capacities such as self-control and intelligence and a more diffuse compassion. Indeed, those who are high in empathy can be too caught up in the suffering of other people. If you absorb the suffering of others, then you're less able to help them in the long run because achieving long-term goals often requires inflicting short-term pain. Any good parent, for instance, often has to make a child do something, or stop doing something, in a way that causes the child immediate unhappiness but is better for him or her in the future: Do your homework, eat your vegetables, go to bed at a reasonable hour, sit still for this vaccination, go to the dentist. Making children suffer temporarily for their own good is made possible by love, intelligence, and compassion, but yet again, it can be impeded by empathy.

I've been focusing here on empathy in the Adam Smith sense, of feeling what others feel and, in particular, feeling their pain. I've argued—and I'll expand on this throughout the rest of the book with more examples and a lot more data—that this sort of empathy is biased and parochial; it focuses you on certain people at the expense of others; and it is innumerate, so it distorts our moral and policy decisions in ways that cause suffering instead of relieving it.

But there is another sense of empathy or, to put it differently, another facet of empathy. There is the capacity to understand what's going on in other people's heads, to know what makes them tick, what gives them joy and pain, what they see as humiliating or ennobling. We're not talking here about me feeling your pain but rather about me understanding that you are in pain without necessarily experiencing any of it myself. Am I against this sort of "cognitive empathy" as well?

I couldn't be. If you see morality in terms of the consequences of our actions—and everyone sees it this way, at least in part—then it follows that being a good moral agent requires an understanding of how people work. How can you ever make people happy if you have no idea what makes them happy? How can you avoid harming people if you don't know what causes them grief? Your intentions might be pure, but if you don't have some grasp of the minds of others, your actions will have, at best, random effects.

If a student is doing poorly and I meet with him to tell him he's failing, it's just basic kindness to try to speak with him in a way that doesn't cause excessive worry or embarrassment. If I'm buying a present for my niece, you don't have to be a moral philosopher to appreciate that I should try to get her something that she wants, not something that I want. To make a positive difference, you need some grasp of what's going on in others' minds.

This sort of understanding is also essential at a policy level.

There has been a lot of debate, for instance, over whether judges should be chosen based in part on their capacity to empathize. Perhaps surprisingly, I think the answer is yes—so long as by *empathy*, one means "cognitive empathy." I agree here with Thomas Colby, who notes that many legal decisions turn on judgments about whether something is cruel or onerous or coerced, and to answer these questions, you need to have some understanding of how people work.

Colby discusses a case involving whether a thirteen-year-old's Fourth Amendment rights were violated by school officials who had her strip-searched because they suspected that she was bringing drugs into the school. Under established doctrine, such a search must be "not excessively intrusive," and Colby notes that judging whether or not this is so involves, in part, knowing what the situation feels like from the standpoint of a thirteen-year-old girl. The judges need cognitive empathy.

But this understanding of the minds of others is an amoral tool, useful for effecting whatever goals you choose. Successful therapists and parents have a lot of cognitive empathy, but so too do successful con men, seducers, and torturers. Or take bullies. There is a stereotype of bullies as social incompetents who take their frustrations out on others. But actually, when it comes to understanding the minds of people, bullies might be better than average—more savvy about what makes other people tick. This is precisely why they can be so successful at bullying. People with low social intelligence, low "cognitive empathy"? Those are more often the bullies' *victims*.

I'll end with a classic fictional example of the power of cognitive empathy. This comes from George Orwell's *1984*—not in the character of the protagonist Winston Smith but in that of

O'Brien, who deceives Winston into thinking of him as a friend but later reveals himself as an agent of the Thought Police and ultimately becomes Winston's torturer.

Orwell's portrayal of O'Brien is fascinating. He is a monster in many ways—Orwell makes him a defender of the cruelest regime imaginable—but he has an easy way with people; he's affable and accessible and excellent at anticipating how others will think and act. When Winston is tortured with electric shock, he feels that his backbone will crack: "'You are afraid,' said O'Brien, watching his face, 'that in another moment something is going to break. Your especial fear is that it will be your backbone. You have a vivid mental picture of the vertebrae snapping apart and the spinal fluid dripping out of them. That is what you are thinking, is it not, Winston?'"

Later O'Brien says, "'Do you remember writing in your diary . . . that it did not matter whether I was a friend or an enemy, since I was at least a person who understood you and could be talked to? You were right. I enjoy talking to you. Your mind appeals to me. It resembles my own mind except that you happen to be insane.'"

Repeatedly, Winston forms a thought and O'Brien goes on to remark on it, apparently reading his mind. Ultimately, O'Brien uses Winston's greatest fear—something he had never told O'Brien, something that he had perhaps never articulated to himself—to destroy him. This is what cognitive empathy looks like in the wrong hands.

Cognitive empathy is a useful tool, then—a necessary one for anyone who wishes to be a good person—but it is morally neutral. I believe that the capacity for emotional empathy, described as "sympathy" by philosophers such as Adam Smith and David Hume, often simply known as "empathy" and defended by so many scholars, theologians, educators, and politicians, is actually morally corrosive. If you are struggling with a moral decision and find yourself trying to feel someone else's pain or pleasure, you should stop. This empathic engagement might give you some satisfaction, but it's not how to improve things and can lead to bad decisions and bad outcomes. Much better to use reason and cost-benefit analysis, drawing on a more distanced compassion and kindness.

The rest of this book will elaborate and qualify this position. It will pull back to explore global politics and zoom in on intimate relationships; it will address the causes of war and the nature of evil. And while I will sometimes concede the benefits of empathy, the verdict is that, on balance, we are better off without it.

There are some perfectly reasonable arguments against this view, many of which might have come to mind during the preceding discussion, and I want to put those objections out here from the start and give quick responses, expanding on most of them in the rest of the book.

The first response brings us back to the terminological issue I raised in the preface.

You say that you're against empathy, but empathy *actually just means kindness, concern, compassion, love, morality, and so on. What you're talking about—trying to feel what others feel—isn't empathy, it's something else.*

I *hate* terminological arguments—nothing important rests on the specific words we use so long as we understand one another. I have a specific notion of empathy in mind, but if you want to reserve the term for something different, there's nothing wrong with that, and if you mean by empathy something like morality, then I'm not against empathy.

But I didn't choose the word at random. The English word *empathy* really is the best way to refer to this mirroring of others' feelings. It's better than *sympathy* (in its modern usage) and *pity*. These terms are only negative; if you are blissfully happy and as a result I feel blissfully happy, I can be said to empathize with you, but it's strange to say that I feel pity for you or sympathy for you. Also, terms like *sympathy* and *pity* are about your reaction to the feelings of others, not the mirroring of them. If you feel bad for someone who is bored, that's sympathy, but if you feel bored, that's empathy. If you feel bad for someone in pain, that's sympathy, but if you feel their pain, that's empathy.

Psychologists have coined the expression "emotional contagion" for situations where the feelings of one person bleed onto another, as when watching someone weep makes you sad or when another's laughter makes you giddy. But while this is related to empathy, it's not quite the same. After all, you can feel empathy when you imagine the plight of someone else, even if there are no emotions in the here and now to catch, and you can feel empathy by inferring another's emotions, even if they aren't actually expressing them.

Finally, empathy is related to *compassion* and *concern*, and sometimes the terms are used synonymously. But compassion and concern are more diffuse than empathy. It is weird to talk about having empathy for the millions of victims of malaria, say, but perfectly normal to say that you are concerned about them or feel compassion for them. Also, compassion and concern don't require mirroring of others' feelings. If someone works to help the victims of torture and does so with energy and good cheer, it doesn't seem right to say that as they do this, they are empathizing with the individuals they are helping. Better to say that they feel compassion for them.

In any case, regardless of how one describes it, we'll see that there are many people who really do think morality is rooted in empathy in the sense that I am discussing here, people who talk about the importance of standing in another's shoes, feeling their pain, and so on. I used to be one of them.

More empathic people are kinder and more caring and more moral. This proves that empathy is a force for good.

Many believe this. After all, to call someone "empathic" (or sometimes "empathetic," but let's not get into *that* argument about words) is a compliment, with empathy probably ranking close to intelligence and a good sense of humor. It's a good thing to put in an online profile for a dating site.

But this claim about the relationship between empathy and certain good traits is an empirical one, something that can be tested using standard psychological methods. For instance, you can measure someone's empathy and then look at whether high empathy predicts good behaviors such as helping others.

Now this is easier said than done. It's hard to accurately measure how empathic a person is. But there have been various efforts, and it turns out that the relationship between empathy and goodness is weak. In fact, we'll see that there is some evidence that high empathy for the suffering of others can paralyze people, lead them to skewed decisions, and often spark irrational cruelty.

People who lack empathy are psychopaths, and those are the worst people in the world. So you need empathy.

Psychopaths do tend to be awful people, and it's also true that, by standard tests, they lack empathy or at least are less willing to deploy it. If it turned out that the first fact follows from the second—that the nastiness associated with psychopathy is due to an empathy deficit—that would be an excellent case for the importance of empathy.

But this is also the sort of thing that you can test in the lab, and it turns out to be unsupported. As we'll see, the problems with psychopaths may have more to do with lack of self-control and a malicious nature than with empathy, and there is little evidence for a relationship between low empathy and being aggressive or cruel to others.

There might be aspects of morality that don't ultimately involve empathy, but empathy is at the core of morality. Without it, there is no justice, fairness, or compassion.

If the claim here is that you need to empathize in order to do good, then it's easy to see that this is mistaken. Think about your judgments about throwing garbage out of your car window, cheating on your taxes, spraying racist graffiti on a building, and similar acts with diffuse consequences. You can appreciate that these are wrong without having to engage in empathic engagement with any specific individuals, real or imagined. Or think about saving a drowning child or giving to a charity. Empathy might be involved there, but it plainly isn't necessary.

Well, the critic concedes, perhaps you can do good things without empathy. But perhaps you can't really care for people — you can't have compassion or concern — without empathy. Psychologists and neuroscientists often make claims such as this: One team of researchers writes, for example, "We can't feel compassion without first feeling emotional empathy," and another claims that "affective empathy is a precursor to compassion."

But, again, it's easy to see that this is a mistake from everyday examples. I see a child crying because she's afraid of a barking dog. I might rush over to pick her up and calm her, and I might really care for her, but there's no empathy there. I don't feel her fear, not in the slightest.

Then there is all the laboratory evidence. We'll see research from the lab of Tania Singer and her colleagues showing that feeling empathy for another person is very different from feeling compassion for that person — distinct in its brain basis and, more important, in its effects. We'll learn about research into the effects of mindfulness meditation suggesting that the boost in kindness that this practice results in part because meditation allows one to stanch one's empathy, not expand it.

But don't you need some sort of emotional push to motivate you to be a good person? Cold reason isn't enough.

"Reason," David Hume famously said, is the "slave of the passions." Good moral deliberation requires valuing some things over others, and good moral action requires some sort of motivational kick in the pants. Even if one knows the best thing to do, one must be motivated to do it.

I believe this—I've never heard a good argument against it. But it's a mistake to see this as an argument for empathy. The "passions" that Hume talks about can be many things. They can be anger, shame, guilt, or, more positively, a more diffuse compassion, kindness, and love. You can be motivated to help others without empathy.

Hume's close friend Adam Smith, that great scholar of the moral sentiments, was aware of this concept. At one point he wonders what motivates us to override our selfish considerations and go to the aid of others. He considers empathy but then rejects it as too weak: "it is not that feeble spark of benevolence which Nature has lifted up in the human heart." Instead he pushes for some combination of careful deliberation and a desire to do the right thing.

Empathy can be used for good. There are cases where our expansion of empathy has led to positive changes. Every moral revolution, from antislavery to gay rights, has used empathy as a spark, and it's used as well in everyday acts of kindness.

I agree with this as well. Empathy can be used to support judgments and actions that, when we reason about them coolly, are morally virtuous. If the right thing to do is to give food to a homeless child, then empathy for the suffering of the child can motivate this giving. If the right thing to do is to expand our moral compass to include members of a once-despised group, empathy for members of that group can bring us there. If the right thing to do is to go to war against another nation, then empathy for the victims of atrocities committed by the nation can motivate the right sort of aggression. Empathy is used as a tool by charitable organizations, religious groups, political parties, and governments, and to the extent that those who spark this empathy have the right moral goals, it can be a valuable force. While I think empathy is a terrible guide to moral judgment, I don't doubt that it can be strategically used to motivate people to do good things.

I have a personal example of this. When I was a graduate student, I read an article by Peter Singer arguing that citizens of prosperous countries should direct most of their money toward helping the truly needy. Singer argued that choosing to spend our money on luxuries like fancy clothing and expensive meals is really no different from seeing a girl drowning in a shallow lake and doing nothing because you don't want to ruin your expensive shoes by wading in to save her. I was moved by this argument and would repeat the analogy to my friends, often when we were in bars and restaurants, and it suddenly occurred to me that we were engaged in the moral equivalent of killing children.

Finally, an exasperated philosophy student asked me how much of my own money I gave to the poor. Embarrassed, I told him the truth: nothing. This weighed on me, so a few days later I sent out a postcard (this was before the Web) to an international aid agency, asking for information as to how I could support their cause.

I remember opening the package they sent me and expecting to see information about what they were up to—statistics and graphs and the like. But they were smarter than that. They sent me a child. A small photograph, wrapped in plastic, of a little boy from Indonesia. I didn't keep the letter they included, but I remember that it went something like this: "We know you haven't committed to giving to our organization. But if you do, this is the life you will save."

I'm not sure if the feeling this prompted was empathy, but it was certainly a sentimental appeal, triggering my heart and not my head. And it worked: Many years later we were still sending money to that child's family.

So, plainly, such sentiments can motivate good behavior. In some cases, it can motivate very good behavior. In Larissa Mac-Farquhar's recent book, *Strangers Drowning*, she talks about the lives of do-gooders or "moral saints." These are people who devote their lives to others. They know that there is immense suffering in the world, and unlike almost everyone else, they can't direct their attention elsewhere; they are driven to help. Some of the individuals she profiles are deliberative and rational, similar to Zell Kravinsky. She talks about Aaron Pitkin, who also read a Singer article and whose life was transformed far more radically than mine: "Nobody would buy a soda if there was a starving child next to the vending machine, he thought; well, for him now there was already a starving child standing next to the vending machine."

But others who are profiled by MacFarquhar are individuals of feeling; they are emotionally moved by the suffering of others. This sensitivity often makes them miserable, but it can also push them to make a difference in ways that most of us would never even contemplate.

Or consider a recent study by Abigail Marsh and her colleagues, of people who choose to donate their kidneys to strangers. Consistent with my argument, these exceptionally altruistic individuals do not score higher on standard empathy tests than normal people. But they are different in another way. The researchers were interested in the amygdala—a part of the brain that is involved in, among other things, emotional responses. Their previous research had discovered that psychopaths had smaller than normal amygdalae and lessened response when exposed to pictures of people who looked frightened, so they predicted that these do-gooders would have larger than normal amygdalae and greater than normal response to fear faces. This was exactly what they found.

What does this mean? One possibility is that these differences in brain anatomy and brain response are the consequence of what kind of person you are—a mind-set of cruelty and exploitation will render you insensitive to the fear of others; a life of kindness and care will make you sensitive to it. Or perhaps these neural differences are causes, not consequences, and your early sensitivity to the suffering of others, which is certainly related to empathy, might influence the sort of person you grow up to be.

One could write a book recounting the good things that arise from empathy. But this is a limited argument in its defense. There are positive effects of just about any strong feeling. Not just empathy but also anger, fear, desire for revenge, and religious fervor—all of these can be used for good causes.

Consider racism. It's easy to think of cases where the worst racist biases are exploited for a good end. Such biases can motivate concern for someone who really does deserve concern, can push one to vote for a politician who really is better than the alternative, can motivate enthusiasm for a war when going to war is the just decision, and so on. But that's not a sufficient argument for racism. One has to show that the good that racism does outweighs the bad and that we are better off using racism to motivate good action rather than alternatives such as compassion and a sense of fairness and justice.

The same holds for empathy. We are often quick to point out the good that empathy does but blind to its costs. I think this is in part because there is a natural tendency to see one's preferred causes and beliefs as bolstered by empathy. That is, people often think about actions that are kind and just (assistance that works, just wars, appropriate punishments) as rooted in empathic feelings, while they view those that are useless or cruel (assistance that fails, unjust wars, brutal punishments) as having other, less empathic sources. But this is an illusion.

Our bias shows up when we think about the power of fiction to stir up our empathy. Many, including myself, have argued that novels like *Uncle Tom's Cabin* and *Bleak House* prompted significant social change by guiding readers to feel the suffering of fictional characters. But we tend to forget that other novels push us in different ways. Joshua Landy provides some examples:

> For every *Uncle Tom's Cabin* there is a *Birth of a Nation*. For every *Bleak House* there is an *Atlas Shrugged*. For every *Color Purple* there is a *Turner Diaries*, that white suprema-

cist novel Timothy McVeigh left in his truck on the way to bombing the Oklahoma building. Every single one of these fictions plays on its readers' empathy: not just high-minded writers like Dickens, who invite us to sympathize with Little Dorrit, but also writers of Westerns, who present poor helpless colonizers attacked by awful violent Native Americans; Ayn Rand, whose resplendent "job-creators" are constantly being bothered by the pesky spongers who merely do the real work; and so on and so on.

Now, one might agree that empathy is on the whole unreliable yet still argue that we should exploit people's empathy for good causes. I have some sympathy with this position, but I worry about the racism analogy. There is good reason to object to appeals to racism even in the service of a good cause because the downside of encouraging this general habit of mind could outweigh whatever good it does in specific cases. I feel the same for empathy and lean toward the view that we should aspire to a world in which a politician appealing to someone's empathy would be seen in the same way as one appealing to people's racist bias.

It's not as if empathy—or emotion more generally—is the only game in town. Landy goes on to defend an alternative, which I think is preferable in many regards:

> The good news is that there are other ways to change people's minds. We can, for example, use the truth. I know, that's very old-fashioned. But consider *An Inconvenient Truth*, Al Gore's documentary about climate change. That film did a huge amount for the environmental movement, all without making up a single lovable character or a single line of witty repar-

tee. Or again, consider *Food, Inc.*, *The Omnivore's Dilemma*, and Jonathan Safran Foer's *Eating Animals*. There haven't been too many meat-industry-themed best-selling fictions in the past hundred years. But that hasn't stopped us as a nation from moving gradually toward more enlightened attitudes.

You've mentioned all sorts of alternatives to empathy. But don't these also suffer from limitations and bias?

They do. I've complained about the problems of empathy, how it works like a spotlight and shines brightest on those we care about. But the other psychological processes involved in moral action and moral judgment are also biased. If you removed our capacity for empathy, somehow excising it from our brains, we would still care more about our families and friends than for strangers. Compassion is biased; concern is biased; and even cost-benefit reasoning is biased. Even when we try hard to be fair, impartial, and objective, we nonetheless tend to tilt things to favor the outcome that benefits ourselves.

But there is a continuum here. On the one extreme is empathy. This is the worst. Then somewhere in the middle is compassion—simply caring for people, wanting them to thrive. This has problems as well but fewer of them, and we'll see that there is experimental evidence—including both neuroimaging studies and research on the effects of meditative practice— suggesting that compassion has some advantages over empathic engagement. In particular, I'll argue that when it comes to certain interpersonal relationships, such as between doctor and patient, compassion is better than empathy. But yes, when it comes to making decisions about charity or war or public policy, many of my arguments against empathy apply to compassion as well.

We do best when we rely on reason. Michael Lynch defines reason as the act of justification and explanation—to provide a reason for something is to justify and explain it, presumably in a way that's convincing to a neutral third party. More specifically, reasoning draws on observation and on principles of logic, with scientific practice being the paradigmatic case of reason at work.

Reason is subject to bias—we are imperfect beings—but at its best it can lead to moral insight. It is reason that leads us to recognize, despite what our feelings tell us, that a child in a faraway land matters as much as our neighbor's child, that it's a tragedy if an immunization leads to a child getting sick or if a furlough program leads to rape and assault—but if these programs nonetheless lead to an overall improvement in human welfare, we should keep them until something better comes along. While sentiments such as compassion motivate us to care about certain ends—to value others and care about doing good—we should draw on this process of impartial reasoning when figuring out how to achieve those ends.

But you just admitted that we're sometimes bad at reasoning. And many psychologists and philosophers would go further and say that we are terrible at it, so much so that we are better off relying on our gut feelings, including empathy.

Our attempts at rational deliberation can get confused or be based on faulty premises or get fogged up by self-interest. But the problem here is with reasoning badly, not with reason itself. We *should* reason our way thorough moral issues. James Rachels sees reason as an essential part of morality—"morality is, at the very least, the effort to guide one's conduct by reason—that is, to do what there are the best reasons for doing—while giving equal weight to the interests of each individual affected by one's decision." Rachels didn't mean this as a psychological claim about how people actually do deal with moral dilemmas but rather as a normative claim about how they should. And I think he's right.

This is less controversial than it sounds. Even the fans of moral emotions implicitly grant priority to reason. If you ask them why they think so highly of empathy (or compassion or pity or anything else), they won't just insist, they won't scream or weep or try to bite you. Rather they'll make *arguments*. They'll talk about positive effects, about the tangible good that these emotions do, about how they align with our most considered priorities. That is, they will defend empathy by appeals to reason.

I don't mean to rag on my colleagues, but there is a certain lack of self-awareness about this point. It is one of the ironies of modern intellectual life that many scholars insist that rationality is impotent, that our efforts at reasoning are at best a smoke screen to justify selfish motivations and irrational feelings. And to make this point, these scholars write books and articles complete with complex chains of logic, citations of data, and carefully reasoned argument. It's like someone insisting that there is no such thing as poetry—and making this case in the form of a poem.

Now, one way my psychologist and philosopher friends might deal with this tension is to claim that most people are incapable of rational deliberation. But they themselves—and those they are writing for, you and me—are the exceptions. We are the special ones who use our heads as well as our hearts. We can think through issues like gay marriage, torture, and so on, while other people are prisoners to their feelings. We have alternatives to emotions like empathy; other people don't.

This is possible, I suppose. But for what it's worth, it doesn't match my own experience. By now I've spoken about moral psychology to many groups of people, not just academics and researchers but high school students and community groups and religious associations. When I do so, I give examples in which empathy pushes us one way and an objective analysis goes another way, as in the Willie Horton case, where our natural feeling for the suffering of his victims might cause us to shut down a program that does more good than harm. Now obviously my audiences don't swoon in agreement when I argue that empathy steers us astray. There is a lot of room for disagreement and counterarguments. But I've never met anyone above the age of seven who didn't appreciate the force of these arguments, agreeing that in certain instances—assuming that I got the facts right—we are better people if we disregard our gut feelings.

To put it differently, I've met people who are stubborn, biased, purposely obtuse, slow on the uptake, suspicious of disagreement, and absurdly defensive—actually, I am very often *exactly* this kind of a person—but I've never met anyone who was insensitive to data and argument in the moral realm and who wasn't capable, at least sometimes, of using moral reasoning to override his or her gut feelings.

We reason best when we have help, and certain communities help reason to flourish. Scientific inquiry is the finest example of how individuals who accept certain practices can work to surpass their individual limitations. Take my attack on empathy, for instance. I really do want to be fair, honest, and objective. But I'm only human, so it's probably true that this book contains weak arguments, cherry-picked data, sneaky rhetorical moves, and unfair representations of those I disagree with. Fortunately, there are many who are in favor of empathy, and they'll be highly motivated to poke holes in my arguments, point out counterevidence, and so on. Then I'll respond, and they'll respond back, and, out of all this, progress will be made.

I'm not starry-eyed about science. Scientists are human, and so we are prone to corruption and groupthink and all sorts of forces that veer us away from the truth. But it does work stunningly well, and this is largely because science provides an excellent example of a community that establishes conditions where rational argument is able to flourish. I think the same holds, to varying extents, in other domains, such as philosophy, the humanities, and even certain sorts of political discourse. We are capable of reason and can exercise this capacity in the domain of morality.

To say that psychological research shows that empathy is a poor moral guide entails some judgments about what's actually right and wrong. This might be worrying. What's a psychologist doing talking about morality anyway?

In my defense, I'm not the one who started this. Most people believe that empathy is a good thing, and many psychologists think that empathy is a *very* good thing, so they write books, have conferences, establish educational programs, and so on, all with the goal of getting people to be more empathic. Plainly I disagree with this, but we share an important premise—which is that there are states of affairs that we should aspire to, outcomes that we should want to achieve. We just disagree about whether empathy is a reliable way of getting to them.

Now I have some moral views that are unusual (I bet you do too), but for the most part I'll try to stick to uncontroversial cases here. So you don't have to agree with my positions on gay marriage or Israel versus Palestine or Kant versus Mill to resonate to my worries about empathy—in fact, I don't think the arguments about empathy connect in any direct way to these specific moral questions. But we do have to agree that it's better (all else being equal) to save a thousand people than just one, that it's wrong to harm someone without cause and wrong to devalue people just because of the color of their skin. If you think numbers don't matter or suffering is good or racism is moral, then many of the arguments that follow will be, at most, of intellectual interest to you.

To the extent that this book is part of a conversation, then it is among people who agree about certain things. To take a specific case, I will argue that our empathy causes us to overrate present costs and underrate future costs. This skews our decisions so that if, say, we are faced with a choice where one specific child will die now or twenty children whose names we don't know will die a year from now, empathy might guide us to choose to save the one. To me, this is a problem with empathy. Now you might respond by saying that this isn't empathy's fault or that empathy might lead us astray here but it's so good in other contexts that we should rely on it more generally. These are legitimate arguments that I will try to address. But if you were instead to say, "So what? Who cares about the death of children?" or "There is no difference between one child dying and twenty children dying," then we don't share enough common ground to proceed.

And so my answer to the question "What does a psychologist have to say about morality?" is: nothing special. But a psychologist might have something to say about the nature of capacities such as empathy and how successful they are at achieving moral ends that we all share. At least that is my hope.

CHAPTER 2

The Anatomy of Empathy

Imagine that you need help. Perhaps you want volunteers for a charity you're running or you're looking for someone strong enough to help you schlep an air conditioner from your car into your apartment. Or maybe it's more serious—suppose your child will die unless you can get enough money from strangers to pay for a lifesaving operation. What could you say that would make people want to help you?

An economist might tell you to try incentives. In the simplest case, you can just pay people—though this plainly won't work if what you need from them is money. Nonmonetary rewards might also work, including those that involve reputation. You don't need laboratory studies to figure out that people are nicer when they know that their actions are public—though, of course, such studies do exist—so one can induce kindness by promising, perhaps in subtle ways, to make these kind actions known to others. That's why certain charities offer mugs or T-shirts to those who donate; these announce the givers' generosity to the world.

Then there is the power of custom. We are social animals,

and our behavior is controlled to a remarkable extent by the behavior of those around us. Even for children, the amount they contribute to someone in need is influenced by what they observe others doing. Another trick to eliciting a certain sort of goodness, then, is to convince people that it's what everyone else is doing.

Sometimes organizations get confused about this, sending out messages that backfire. I was once in a dining hall at the University of Chicago and saw a sign: "Do you realize that more than 1,000 dishes and utensils are taken from this dining commons each quarter?" Presumably the intention of the sign was to shock the students into compliance—that's terrible, I didn't know it was so bad, I'd never do that!—but for me, at least, the effect was to make me want to slip a knife and fork into my jacket pocket. If you want people to stop doing something, don't tell them that everyone does it.

Incentives appeal to self-interest, custom appeals to our social nature, but a third way to elicit kindness is to get people to feel empathy. Much of the best research here comes from the laboratory of C. Daniel Batson. In a typical study, Batson and his colleagues put subjects in a situation where they have the opportunity to do something nice—such as donating money, taking over an unpleasant task from someone else, or cooperating with someone at a cost. Some of the subjects are told nothing or are told to take an objective point of view. But others are encouraged to feel empathy—they might be told: "Try to take the other person's perspective" or "Put yourself in that person's shoes."

Over and over again, Batson finds that these empathy prompts make subjects more likely to do good—to give money, take over a task, and cooperate. Empathy makes them kind.

Batson finds these effects even when helping is anonymous, when there is a justification for not helping, and when it's easy to say no. He concludes from his work that these effects cannot be explained by a desire to enhance one's reputation or a wish to avoid embarrassment or anything like that. Rather, empathy elicits a genuine desire to make another person's life better.

These are robust findings, and they make intuitive sense. Suppose you really were face-to-face with someone who, with some sacrifice on his part, could save your dying child. Your first move might be to elicit empathy, to get the person to feel your child's pain or perhaps your own. Your first words might be: "How would you feel if it were your child?"

Charities do this sort of thing all the time, using pictures and stories to get you to empathize with suffering people. I once told the leader of a charitable organization that I was writing a book encouraging people to be less empathic, and she got angry, telling me that if she couldn't stir up empathy, her group would get less money, and then some of the children she had spent so much time with would die.

Let's put aside the issue of charity for now—I promise to return to it in the next chapter—and step back to marvel at empathy's power. It's like magic. Let's see now what sort of magic it is.

Nowadays, many people only seriously consider claims about our mental lives if you can show them pretty pictures from a brain scanner. Even among psychologists who should know better, images derived from PET or fMRI scans are seen as reflecting something more scientific—more *real*—than anything else a psychologist could discover. There is a particular obsession with localization, as if knowing where something is in the brain is the key to explaining it.

I see this when I give popular talks. The question I dread most is "Where does it happen in the brain?" Often, whoever asks this question knows nothing about neuroscience. I could make up a funny-sounding brain part—"It's in the flurbus murbus"—and my questioner would be satisfied. What's really wanted is some reassurance that there is true science going on and that the phenomenon I'm discussing actually exists. To some, this means that I have to say something specific about the brain.

This assumption reflects a serious confusion about the mind and how to study it. After all, unless one is a neuroanatomist, the brute facts about specific location—that the posterior cingulate gyrus is active during certain sorts of moral deliberation, say— are, in and of themselves, boring. Moral deliberation has to be *somewhere* in the brain, after all. It's not going to be in the foot or the stomach, and it's certainly not going to reside in some mysterious immaterial realm. So who cares about precisely where?

But while localization itself is a snooze, it's clear by now that the tools of neuroscience, properly applied, can give us considerable insight into how the mind works. There is currently a lot of excitement about "social neuroscience"—or sometimes "affective neuroscience"—and much of it is deserved.

To study empathy, neuroscientists use diverse and clever methods. In the typical experiment, subjects are given some sort of experience. They might be shown pictures of people's faces or hands, or movies that depict different activities or emotional reactions; they might be made to feel mild pain or watch someone else feel mild pain; they might be told a story or asked to take a particular attitude toward a person or situation, such as being objective or empathic.

In many of the studies, the subject's brain is scanned during the experience, though other approaches are sometimes taken. Recent research, for instance, involves zapping the brain with electromagnetic energy—transcranial magnetic stimulation— to see what happens when certain areas are stimulated or dulled. And there is a long tradition of studying individuals with brain injuries to see what impairments are associated with specific sorts of damage.

What these studies do, in essence, is find out what parts of the brain are involved in what activities (and also, sometimes, what the time course of mental processes is—the order in which the brain areas are activated). This is the sort of localization I was disparaging, but it doesn't end there. The best studies go on to compare and contrast the correlates of mental activity to tell us what aspects of mental life fall together and what influences what.

If you're one of those people who doesn't believe something is real unless you see it in the brain, you'll be relieved to hear that empathy actually does exist. It really does light up the brain. Actually, at first blush, empathy looks as if it's *everywhere* in the brain. One scholar describes at length what he calls "an empathy circuit in the brain," but this "circuit" contains ten major brain areas, some of them big chunks of brain stuff, larger than a baby's finger, like the medial prefrontal cortex, the anterior insula, and the amygdala—all of which are also engaged in actions and experiences that have nothing to do with empathy.

It turns out, though, that this the-whole-brain-does-it conclusion arises because neuroscientists—along with psychologists and philosophers—are often sloppy in their use of the term *empathy*. Some investigators look at what I see as empathy proper— what happens in the brain when someone feels the same thing they believe another person is feeling. Others look at what happens when we try to understand other people, usually called "social cognition" or "theory of mind" but sometimes called "cognitive empathy." Others look at quite specific instantiations of empathy (such as what happens when you watch someone's face contort in disgust), and still others study what goes on in the brain when a person decides to do something nice for another person, which is sometimes called "prosocial concern" but which one normally thinks of as niceness or kindness. Once you start pulling these different phenomena apart, which I'll do below, things get more interesting, and you see how these different capacities relate to one another.

After many years and many millions of dollars, it turns out that there are three major findings from the neuroscience of empathy research. None of these are exactly new—they reinforce ideas from philosophers hundreds of years ago—but they add to our knowledge in valuable ways.

The first finding is that an empathic response to someone else's experience can involve the same brain tissue that's active when you yourself have that experience. So "I feel your pain" isn't just a gooey metaphor; it can be made neurologically literal: Other people's pain really does activate the same brain area as your own pain, and more generally, there is neural evidence for a correspondence between self and other.

One of the best-known findings along these lines emerged about fifteen years ago from the lab of Giacomo Rizzolatti, in Italy. The scientists had parts of the premotor cortex of pigtail macaque monkeys wired up so as to record neural activity when the monkeys engaged in certain actions. They then discovered that these same neural responses sometimes occurred when the monkeys weren't overtly doing anything at all but just watching the scientists in the laboratory grasp and manipulate objects. Certain neurons, then, didn't appear to distinguish between an action-the-monkey-does and an action-the-monkey-perceives-someone-else-doing. Fittingly, these became known as "mirror neurons."

One modest theory of the function of these mirror neurons is that they help solve the problem of how monkeys figure out how to manipulate objects. That is, given their mirroring properties, these neurons could help the monkey calibrate his or her own grip based on observing what others do. But for Rizzolatti and his colleagues, this was just the beginning. They, and soon many others, began to explore mirror neurons as a theory of how we can understand the mental states of other individuals, and soon proposed them as part of a theory of empathy. After all, a neural system that doesn't make the distinction between self and other seems tailor-made for explaining how we can share the experiences of others.

Mirror neurons have a lot of fans. One prominent neuroscientist said that they will do for psychology what DNA did for biology—another described them as "tiny miracles that get us through the day." Godwin's Law says that as any online discussion proceeds, the odds of someone mentioning Hitler approaches certainty. In my experience, there is an equivalent for mirror neurons. In any discussion of some psychological capacity (including empathy), you don't have to wait long until someone reminds the group that we already have a perfectly good theory—it's all done by mirror neurons.

In his book *The Myth of Mirror Neurons*, Gregory Hickok notes that if you google "mirror neurons" you will learn about gay mirror neurons, how the president is using mirror neurons to peek into your brain, why God created mirror neurons to make us better people, and much else. His survey of scientific journal articles finds that mirror neurons are said to be implicated in (just to take a selection) stuttering, schizophrenia, hypnosis, cigarette smoking, obesity, love, business leadership, music appreciation, political attitudes, and drug abuse.

As you might be able to tell from the title of his book, Hickok is critical of the claims that have been made about mirror neurons, and many scholars would agree that they have been overhyped. One strong objection to the view that they explain capacities such as morality, empathy, and language is that most of the findings about mirror neurons come from macaque monkeys—and monkeys don't have much morality, empathy, or language. Mirror neurons cannot be sufficient for these capacities, then—though they might help out with them.

Nevertheless, the more general finding of shared representations—the discovery that there exist neural systems that treat the experiences and actions of others the same way they treat the experiences and actions of the self—really is an important discovery about mental life.

Most of the research along these lines has focused on pain. Several studies find that certain parts of the brain—including the anterior insula and the cingulate cortex—are active both when you feel pain and when you watch someone else feel pain. The pain that the subject is made to experience can be an electric shock or a pinprick to the finger, a blast of noise through headphones or the application of heat—what one study carefully described as "painful thermal stimulation"—administered to the subject's left hand. The pain of the other person can be conveyed by having the subjects watch the other person being shocked, pricked, blasted, or baked; by having them just look at the person's face while this is happening; or even just by providing them with a written description of the event. While almost all of these studies are done with adults, there are similar results for children. And no matter how you test it, there is neural overlap; the neural expression of the observed pain of the other is similar to what you would get if you yourself were in pain.

Other research looks at disgust. A part of the brain known as the anterior insula (which is also involved in pain, among other things) lights up both when you feel disgusted and when you look at someone else being disgusted. There is something intuitive about this finding. Many years ago there was a particularly vivid viral video, called "2 girls, 1 cup," which I'm not going to describe here, except to say that it really was extremely disgusting. (If you're tempted to look for it online, consider this a trigger warning.) The online magazine Slate had the interesting idea of showing a video of people watching the video, so you can see their faces contort as they respond. The face video is hilarious, but also disgusting—watching the disgust of others triggers a hint of disgust in yourself.

You can see this overlap between self and other as a clever evolutionary trick. To thrive as a social being, one has to make sense of the internal lives of other individuals, to accurately guess what other people are thinking, wanting, and feeling. Since we're not telepathic, we have to infer this from information we get from our senses. One possible solution is that we come to understand people in the same way that we come to understand any other phenomenon, like the growth of plants or the movement of stars in the night sky. But there's an alternative. We can take advantage of the fact that we have minds ourselves, and we can use our own minds as a laboratory to bring ourselves up to speed on how others will behave and think.

To see how this works, answer this: Which English word is someone more likely to know the meaning of—*fish* or *transom*? You could try to answer this by thinking about how common the words are, the circumstances under which one is likely to learn them, how often they show up in everyday speech, and so on. But there's a better way. What you probably did when answering this question was to quickly judge which word was easier for *you* to understand and then assume that others would be just like you. You used yourself as a lab rat to make inferences about others.

We can do the same for subjective experiences. Which would hurt a stranger more: stubbing her toe or slamming her hand in a car door? You could try to figure this out from scratch, like a scientist looking at the biological workings of a novel species, but a better way is to assess memories of your own pain (or just to imagine yourself in those situations) and assume that the other person will feel the same way you do.

This sort of simulation has its limits, though. It assumes that others are similar to you—an assumption that is sometimes mistaken. Many people believe that dogs enjoy being hugged, for example, presumably because *we* enjoy being hugged. But this is probably wrong: Dog experts tell us that dogs don't naturally enjoy being hugged; they suffer through it. A lot of misery in the world—and a lot of bad birthday presents—exists because we understand other people by using ourselves as a model: This doesn't offend me, so I assume it doesn't offend you. I like this, so I assume you do too. And sometimes we get it wrong. As the Latin maxim goes, *De gustibus non est disputandum.*

Our occasional success at understanding individuals who are different from ourselves shows that simulation can't be the whole story in understanding other people. Hickok points out that we can often successfully read the minds of dogs and cats, figure out what they mean when they bark or purr, wag their tails, put their tails up high, and so on, but surely we're not simulating them. Those who are quadriplegic from birth can have a rich understanding of other people, figuring out their mental states based on their movement—she has loudly slammed the door, she must be angry—even though these quadriplegics are not in any sense simulating the actions. And I can appreciate that other people will enjoy cheese, though I hate it myself, just as I can be good at buying presents for two-year-olds, though they are rarely the sorts of gifts that I myself would like. We can transcend simulation when appreciating the minds of others.

Finally, we shouldn't exaggerate the extent to which we mirror others. The neuroscience evidence shows an overlap, but it also shows differences. You can look at an fMRI scan and tell the difference between someone being poked in the hand and someone watching another person being poked in the hand. And, of course, there has to be a brain difference between self and other because there is a psychological difference. Watching someone getting slapped in the face doesn't really make your cheek burn, and watching someone get a back rub doesn't make your aches go away. We may feel the pain of someone else, in a limited sense, but in another sense we really don't. Relative to real experience, empathic resonance is pallid and weak.

Even without access to an fMRI scanner, Adam Smith made the same point hundreds of years ago, pointing out that empathic experience is not just different in degree but in kind. Our appreciation that this experience isn't really happening to us "not only lowers it in degree, but, in some measure, varies it in kind, and gives it a quite different modification."

An empathic response can be automatic and rapid. If you see someone hitting his finger with a hammer, you might flinch, and this seems to be a reflexive response. But for the most part, whether or not we are consciously aware of it, empathy is modified by our beliefs, expectations, motivations, and judgments. This is the second finding from neuroscience: Our empathic experience is influenced by what we think about the person we are empathizing with and how we judge the situation that person is in.

It turns out, for instance, that you feel more empathy for someone who treats you fairly than for someone who has cheated you. And you feel more empathy for someone who is cooperating with you than for someone you are in competition with. Or take a study where subjects were shown videos of people in pain, said to be suffering from AIDS. Some of these individuals were described as having been infected through intravenous drug use, while others were described as getting AIDS through a blood transfusion. People said that they felt less empathy for the person who became infected through drug use—and their neural activation told the same story: When they viewed this individual, they had less activation in brain areas associated with pain, such as, again, the anterior cingulate cortex. And the more subjects explicitly blamed the drug users for their fate, the less empathy they said they had and the less brain activation there was.

Again, Adam Smith was here first, observing that the empathy we feel toward others is sensitive to all sorts of considerations. He notes that you're not going to feel an empathically positive response toward someone who has a sudden and great success—envy blocks this sort of pleasure. And you're not going to feel the pain of those whose problems you see as their own fault or that you view as insignificant. It's hard to feel empathy for whiners. Smith gives the example of a man who is really annoyed because while he was telling a story to his brother, his brother was humming. You're not going to empathize with *that*, Smith points out. You're more likely to find it funny.

Empathy is also influenced by the group to which the other individual belongs—whether the person you are looking at or thinking about is one of Us or one of Them. One European study tested male soccer fans. The fan would receive a shock on the back of his hand and then watch another man receive the same shock. When the other man was described as a fan of the subject's team, the empathic neural response—the overlap in self-other pain—was strong. But when the man was described as a fan of the opposing team, it wasn't.

Or consider the response to those who repel us. Lasana Harris and Susan Fiske got subjects to view pictures of drug addicts and homeless people. Subjects found these pictures to be disgusting and showed correspondingly reduced activity in the medial prefrontal cortex, a chunk of the brain involved in social reasoning. Although this study didn't directly look at empathy, the findings do suggest that we shut off our social understanding when dealing with certain people: We dehumanize them.

We see how reactions to others, including our empathic reactions, reflect prior bias, preference, and judgment. This shows that it can't be that empathy simply makes us moral. It has to be more complicated than that because whether or not you feel empathy depends on prior decisions about who to worry about, who counts, who matters—and these are moral choices. Your empathy doesn't drive your moral evaluation of the drug user with AIDS. Rather it's your moral evaluation of the person that determines whether or not you feel empathy.

The third important finding from neuroscience concerns the difference between feeling and understanding.

I've been using the term *empathy* in the sense of Adam Smith's *sympathy*—feeling what another feels. But one can ask how this sharing of feelings relates to the ability to understand people's psychological states. I've repeatedly pointed out that we sometimes call this *empathy* as well—"cognitive empathy"—and one might wonder whether they are one and the same.

If they were, it would call into question my argument against empathy. You can't make it through life without some capacity to understand the minds of others. So if feeling the pain of others arises from the same neural system that underlies everyday social understanding—if you can't have one without the other—then giving up on emotional empathy would be giving up too much.

Some scholars do put the two together, talking about "projective empathy" in a way that doesn't distinguish between understanding and feeling. And one popular metaphor, that of putting yourself in another person's shoes, lumps together knowing what someone thinks and feeling what someone feels.

Still, talk about projection, or shoe-sharing, is just metaphor. What really happens when you deal with other people is that you get information through your senses (you see their facial expressions, you hear what they are saying, and so on), and this information influences what you believe and what you feel. One way it can influence you is by informing you about the mental states of the other person (you believe *she is in pain*); another way it can influence you is by causing you to have certain feelings (you feel pain yourself). Now, it's certainly possible that one neural system does both of these things and that understanding and shared feelings have a common source. But it's also possible that these are two separate processes and, importantly, that you can understand that someone is in pain without actually feeling it.

In fact, the separate processes theory seems to be the right one. In a review article, Jamil Zaki and Kevin Ochsner note that hundreds of studies now support a certain perspective on the mind, which they call "a tale of two systems." One system involves sharing the experience of others, what we've called empathy; the other involves inferences about the mental states of others—mentalizing or mind reading. While they can both be active at once, and often are, they occupy different parts of the brain. For instance, the medial prefrontal cortex, just behind the forehead, is involved in mentalizing, while the anterior cingulate cortex, sitting right behind that, is involved in empathy.

This separateness has some interesting consequences. Consider how to make sense of criminal psychopaths. One recent scientific article struggles with the question of whether these troubling individuals are high in empathy or low in empathy. For the authors, the evidence suggests both: "Psychopathic criminals can be charming and attuned while seducing a victim, thereby suggesting empathy, and later callous while raping a victim, thereby suggesting impaired empathy." So which is it?

The authors try to resolve this apparent paradox in terms of a distinction between ability (one's capacity to deploy empathy) and propensity (one's willingness to do so). They suggest that these criminal psychopaths have normal empathic ability but adjust it like the dial of a radio—turn it up when you want to listen to the lyrics, turn it down if you want to focus on passing a slow truck on the I-95. Turn up empathy when you want to figure out how to charm people and win their trust; turn it down when you're assaulting them.

They're surely right that this distinction exists: Two individuals can have the same capacity for empathy but choose to deploy it to different extents, and we've already seen that empathy can be triggered or stanched by your relationship with the person you're dealing with. And maybe that's partially what's going on with the criminal psychopaths.

But the neuroscience research tells us that there's a simpler analysis. The mental life of the psychopath is only a puzzle if you think that the ability to make sense of people's mental states (useful for charming someone) is the same as the ability to feel other's experiences, including their pain (which gets in the way of assaulting someone). But they aren't. So criminal psychopaths don't have to be fiddling with a single dial of empathy: A simpler explanation is that they are good at understanding other people and bad at feeling their pain. They have high cognitive empathy but low emotional empathy.

None of this is to deny that understanding and feeling are related. Smell, vision, and taste are separate, but they come together in the appreciation of a meal, and it might be that the act of adopting someone's perspective in a cold-blooded way makes you more likely to vicariously experience what they are feeling and vice versa. But these are nonetheless different processes, and this is important to keep in mind when we think about the pros and cons of empathy.

The research we just talked about takes empathy down a peg. We mirror the feelings of others, but this mirroring is limited: Empathic suffering is different from actual suffering. Empathy is also contingent on how one feels about an individual. It's not always the case, then, that we feel empathy and thereby treat someone well. Instead, we often think that someone is worth treating kindly (because he or she treated us nicely in the past or is simply like us) and *then* we feel empathy. And finally, emotional empathy—the sort of empathy that we're obsessing about here—can be usefully disentangled from the essential capacity of understanding other people.

But we cannot forget where we started, which is the experimental research on the powers of empathy. In the laboratory, and sometimes in the real world, empathy makes us better people. This is the magic we have to explain.

Why would empathy make us nicer? The obvious answer— the one that comes to mind immediately for many people—is that empathy allows our selfish motivations to extend to others. The clearest case of this is when someone else's pain is experienced as your own pain. The idea is that you will help because this will make your own pain go away. This view is nicely expressed by Jean-Jacques Rousseau, in *Emile, or On Education*: "But if the enthusiasm of an overflowing heart identifies me with my fellow-creature, if I feel, so to speak, that I will not let him suffer lest I should suffer too, I care for him because I care for myself, and the reason of the precept is found in nature herself, which inspires me with the desire for my own welfare wherever I may be."

This theory has the advantage of simplicity, as it explains the moral power of empathy in terms of the obvious fact that nobody (well, almost nobody) likes to suffer. It suggests that empathic motivations are, in the end, selfish ones.

It's not clear, though, that selfishness can explain the good acts that empathy leads to. When empathy makes us feel pain, the reaction is often a desire to escape. Jonathan Glover tells of a woman who lived near the death camps in Nazi Germany and who could easily see atrocities from her house, such as prisoners being shot and left to die. She wrote an angry letter: "One is often an unwilling witness to such outrages. I am anyway sickly and such a sight makes such a demand on my nerves that in the long run I cannot bear this. I request that it be arranged that such inhuman deeds be discontinued, or else be done where one does not see it."

She was definitely suffering from seeing the treatment of the prisoners, but it didn't motivate her to want to save them: She would be satisfied if she could have this suffering continue out of her sight. This feeling shouldn't be that alien to many of us. People often cross the street to avoid encountering suffering people who are begging for money. It's not that they don't care (if they didn't care, they would just walk by), it's that they are bothered by the suffering and would rather not encounter it. Usually, escape is even easier. Steven Pinker writes: "For many years a charity called Save the Children ran magazine ads with a heartbreaking photograph of a destitute child and the caption 'You can save Juan Ramos for five cents a day. Or you can turn the page.' Most people turn the page."

A final example is fictional, from H. G. Wells's *The Island of Doctor Moreau*. The narrator, Edward Prendick, is disturbed by the screaming of a suffering animal: "It was as if all the pain in the world had found a voice. Yet had I known such pain was in the next room, and had it been dumb, I believe—I have thought since—I could have stood it well enough. It is when suffering finds a voice and sets our nerves quivering that this pity comes troubling us."

This has been cited as an example of the moral force of felt experience and the power of empathy. But what does Prendick do? He *leaves*. He goes for a walk to escape the noise, finds a space in the shade, and takes a nap.

So if vicarious suffering were the sole outcome of empathy, empathy would be mostly useless as a force for helping others. There is almost always an easier way to make your empathic suffering go away than the hard work of making someone else's life better: Turn the page. Look away. Cover your ears. Think of something else. Take a nap.

To the extent that empathy drives us to do positive things for others in situations where there are easy escapes, it must be motivating us in a different way. Indeed, some of the clever experiments developed by Batson and his colleagues gave people the option to leave the study—but they typically don't take this option. Instead they help the person they are feeling empathy for. This is an embarrassment for the selfish-motivation theory.

I favor Batson's own analysis that empathy's power lies in its capacity to make the experience of others observable and salient, therefore harder to ignore. If I love my baby, and she's in anguish, empathy with her pain will make me pick her up and try to make her pain go away. This is not because doing so makes *me* feel better—it does, but if I just wanted my vicarious suffering to go away, I'd leave the crying baby and go for a walk. Rather, my empathy lets me know that someone I love is suffering, and since I love her, I'll try to make her feel better.

This is a different perspective on why empathic appeals so often work. It's not that empathy itself automatically leads to kindness. Rather, empathy has to connect to kindness that already exists. Empathy makes good people better, then, because kind people don't like suffering, and empathy makes this suffering salient. If you made a sadist more empathic, it would just lead to a happier sadist, and if I were indifferent to the baby's suffering, her crying would be nothing more than an annoyance.

Empathy can also support broader moral principles. If someone were to slap me, it would be unpleasant, physically and psychologically. This in itself won't make me realize that it's wrong for me to slap other people. But if I feel empathy for those who are slapped—if I can appreciate that it feels to them the way it feels to me—this can help me arrive at a generalization: If the slapping is wrong when it happens to me, it might well be wrong when it happens to someone else.

In this way, empathy can help you appreciate that you are not special. It's not only that I don't want to be slapped, it's also that *he* doesn't want to be slapped, and *she* doesn't want to be slapped, and so on. This can support the generalization that nobody wants to be slapped, which can in turn support a broader prohibition against slapping. In this regard, empathy and morality can be mutually reinforcing: The exercise of empathy makes us realize that we are not special after all, which supports the notion of impartial moral principles, which motivates us to continue to empathize with other people.

For someone who is a fan of empathy, this is a start at explaining why it is a force for good.

This is how the magic works, how empathy can do good. But what are its actual effects in the real world? One way to try to answer this is to look at the relationship between how empathic and how moral a person is. Are empathic people morally better, on average, than less empathic people?

As you might imagine, there has been a lot of work on this question. But before getting to the findings, it's worth noting that this is difficult research to do well. It's hard to measure the good that people do, how moral they are. And it's hard to measure how empathic people are.

Let's zoom in on the measurement problem. Some people are more empathic than others. They are more prone to feel what others are feeling. In principle, there are a lot of ways to test where any individual lies on the continuum. These include subtle methods such as those described above, like assessing brain activation in the neural areas associated with empathy. But such methods are expensive and difficult. So most large-scale experiments assess empathy the same way that they assess narcissism or anxiety or open-mindedness or any of the other traits psychologists are interested in—they ask a series of questions. Researchers use responses to these questions to get a score for each person, and then they see how this score relates to something associated with goodness or badness, which is itself assessed through observation or experiment or by asking yet more questions.

Administering questionnaires is easier than other methods, but it has its problems. For one, it's hard to tell whether you are measuring actual empathy as opposed to how much people see themselves or want others to see them as empathic. To put it crudely, some people who aren't actually empathic might believe they are or want others to believe they are and answer accordingly.

Another problem is that these studies rarely factor out other aspects of individuals that might well correlate with high empathy, such as intelligence, self-control, and a broader compassionate worldview. By analogy, children with excellent teeth are more likely to get into elite universities than children with bad teeth; any study would find a correlation. But it would be a mistake to say that the teeth themselves are relevant—dentistry is not destiny. Rather, children with excellent teeth are likely to have richer parents and grow up in better environments and so on, and it's these other, more significant factors that actually explain the correlation. Similarly, it might not be empathy driving any good effects but rather certain personality traits that are associated with empathy.

Another issue is that the standard empathy scales are imperfect measures of empathy. The most popular measures include questions that are related to empathy in the sense of mirroring others' feelings, but they also have questions that tap other capacities, such as kindness or compassion or interest in others.

Take as an example the well-known scale developed by Mark Davis and used by many scholars—including me and my students in unrelated work on belief in fate. It contains four parts, with seven items each, developed so that each can tap, as Davis puts it, "a separate aspect of the global concept, 'empathy.'" The scales include *Perspective Taking*, tailored to capture people's interest in taking the perspectives of others; *Fantasy*, their tendency to identify with fictional characters; *Empathic Concern*, which focuses on feelings for others; and *Personal Distress*, which measures how much anxiety people feel when they observe others' negative experiences.

The *Fantasy* scale includes the following items—for each, you're supposed to rate yourself on a scale running from "does not describe me well" to "describes me very well":

- When I am reading an interesting story or novel, I imagine how I would feel if the events in the story were happening to me.
- I really get involved with the feelings of the characters in a novel.
- I daydream and fantasize, with some regularity, about things that might happen to me.

These items do well in assessing an appetite for fictional engagement. But this is separate from what we're interested in here: Someone might have high empathy but not care much about fiction, or have low empathy but love to daydream and fantasize.

The *Perspective Taking* scale does involve some empathy-related items, but it also explores the presence of a certain open-minded attitude when it comes to disagreements. The items include:

- I believe that there are two sides to every question and try to look at them both.
- I try to look at everybody's side of a disagreement before I make a decision.

Again, one can score high on both of these items without being in the slightest bit empathic, not even in a cognitive empathy sense. Or one can score low on these items but be highly empathic in every other sense.

The last two scores—*Empathic Concern* and *Personal Distress*—are seen by many as reflecting the core of empathy. But these scales don't adequately distinguish between feeling others' pain and simply caring about other people. Items on the *Empathic Concern* scale, for instance, include:

- I am often quite touched by things that I see happen.
- Sometimes I don't feel sorry for other people when they are having problems. (reverse coded: low score = high empathic concern)
- I care for my friends a great deal.
- I feel sad when I see a lonely stranger in a group.

These certainly tap something morally relevant about a person. But it's not necessarily how prone they are to feel empathy; rather, it's how much they care about other people.

The *Personal Concern* scale has deeper problems because it basically measures how likely you are to lose your cool in an emergency. Items include:

- When I see someone who badly needs help in an emergency, I go to pieces.
- In emergency situations, I feel apprehensive and ill-at-ease.
- I tend to lose control during emergencies.

Now this might have *something* to do with empathy. Perhaps highly empathic people are more likely to get upset during a crisis. But the connection with empathy is uncertain, particularly since it's not made clear that the emergencies have to do with the suffering of others. Someone might freak out when a sewer pipe bursts or when there's a tornado coming down the road, but this has nothing to do with empathy—or with compassion or altruism or anything like that.

Another popular scale is the *Empathy Quotient*, which was developed by Simon Baron-Cohen and Sally Wheelwright in the context of Baron-Cohen's influential "empathizing-systemizing" theory. Baron-Cohen claims that, on average, women are higher on empathizing and men are higher on systematizing—an interest in analyzing or constructing systems. Individuals with autism are seen as possessing "extreme male brains," with an unusual focus on systematizing, which is often reflected in an obsessive focus on domains such as train schedules and jigsaw puzzles, and lower levels of empathizing, which is partially responsible for their difficulties in relating to others.

I think Baron-Cohen's theory is interesting, but the scale that he uses to tap "empathizing" is a hodgepodge. Some questions do perfectly capture empathy, such as:

- I find it easy to put myself in somebody else's shoes.
- Seeing people cry doesn't really upset me." (reverse coded)

But others tap a form of social adroitness that has little to do with either empathy or compassion:

- I can easily tell if someone else wants to enter a conversation.
- People often tell me that I went too far in driving my point home in a discussion. (reverse coded)
- I find it hard to know what to do in a social situation. (reverse coded)

Baron-Cohen does research on autism, and his scale seems oriented toward capturing certain features that are characteristic of individuals with this condition. But it's not adequate as an empathy scale. After all, someone could be highly empathic but socially awkward, or socially skilled without being empathic at all.

It turns out, then, that all the empathy measures that are commonly used are actually measures of a cluster of things—including empathy, but also concern and compassion, as well as some traits, such as being cool-headed in an emergency, that might have little to do with empathy in any sense of the term.

Finally, when it comes to looking at research concerning the relationship between empathy and good behavior, there is the issue of publication bias. Researchers who study the effects of empathy are typically hoping and expecting that empathy does have effects—nobody does an experiment hoping to find nothing. Studies that fail to find an effect are therefore less likely to be submitted for publication (the so-called file drawer problem), and if such work is submitted, it's more difficult to get published, because null effects are notoriously uninteresting to reviewers and editors.

All these problems—biases in self-report, the fact that other traits might correlate with high empathy, problems with the scales, and biases in publication—would lead to published studies inflating the relationship between empathy and good behavior. So what is the relationship?

Surprisingly, even given all these considerations in favor of finding an effect, there isn't much of one. There have been hundreds of studies, with children and adults, and overall the results are: meh. Some studies find some small relationship; others find none or yield uncertain and mixed findings. There are meta-analyses that put together studies to see what the big picture is, and some of these come to the conclusion that there is no effect of empathy and others that there is one, but it's weak and hard to find. (As always, if you want to see citations of actual studies and meta-analyses, check out the endnotes.) The biggest effect of empathy occurs with the Batson experimental studies I've discussed earlier, where empathy is induced in the laboratory. Studies that look at individual differences using questionnaires find much less of an effect.

I've been talking about the association between high empathy and good behavior. But what if you turned it around and looked at the low end of the spectrum—not at whether high empathy makes you good but at whether low empathy makes you bad? What about the relationship between low empathy and aggression?

I'm an empathy skeptic like no other, but even I think there should be some relationship between being low in empathy and being prone to violent and cruel behavior. It makes sense that empathy inhibits cruelty. If I feel your pain, I'm less likely to cause it in the first place because it hurts me. Individuals with low empathy don't have such a force inhibiting them, so there should be some correlation between being low in empathy and being badly behaved.

But here, at least, I'm giving empathy too much credit. A recent paper reviewed the findings from all available studies of the relationship between empathy and aggression. The results are summarized in the title: "The (Non)Relation between Empathy and Aggression: Surprising Results from a Meta-Analysis." They report that only about 1 percent of the variation in aggression is accounted for by lack of empathy. This means that if you want to predict how aggressive a person is, and you have access to an enormous amount of information about that person, including psychiatric interviews, pen-and-paper tests, criminal records, and brain scans, the last thing you would bother to look at would be measures of the person's empathy.

The authors plainly didn't expect this, and they spend much of the conclusion of the paper puzzling over their odd finding—or more precisely, their odd lack of finding. They end up concluding that it suggests that we take empathy too seriously. They note that when we think of a low-empathy person, we think of a callous, unemotional person who cares little about the welfare of others. But this is mistaken. As they put it, "There are emotions and considerations outside of empathy, and there are many reasons to care about others."

Being high in empathy doesn't make one a good person, and being low in empathy doesn't make one a bad person. What we'll see in the chapters that follow is that goodness might be related to more distanced feelings of compassion and care, while evil might have more to do with a lack of compassion, a lack of regard for others, and an inability to control one's appetites.

CHAPTER 3

Doing Good

One of the best arguments in favor of empathy is that it makes you kinder to the person you are empathizing with. This is backed by laboratory research, by everyday experience, and by common sense. So if the world were a simple place, where the only dilemmas one had to deal with involved a single person in some sort of immediate distress, and where helping that person had positive effects, the case for empathy would be solid.

But the world is not a simple place. Often—very often, I will argue—the action that empathy motivates is not what is morally right.

Most laboratory studies don't tap this complexity. The experiments are designed to measure the effects of empathy in terms of some action that is plainly good—more helping, more cooperation, more kindness toward an individual who plainly needs help. But there is one significant exception, a clever study done by C. Daniel Batson and his colleagues.

Now, Batson has defended the "empathy-altruism hypothesis"— the idea that empathy motivates the helping of others—but he does not claim that empathy inevitably has positive consequences.

As he puts it, "Empathy-induced altruism is neither moral nor immoral; it is amoral."

To explore this, he set up a situation in which empathy pushed people toward an answer that most people would believe, upon consideration, is the wrong one. He told his subjects about a charitable organization called the Quality Life Foundation that worked to make the final years of terminally ill children more comfortable. The subjects were then told that they would hear interviews with individual children on the waiting list for treatment. Subjects in the low-empathy condition were told: "While you are listening to this interview, try to *take an objective perspective toward what is described.* Try not to get caught up in how the child who is interviewed feels; just remain objective and detached." And those in the high-empathy condition were told: "Try to imagine how the child who is interviewed feels about what has happened and how it has affected this child's life. Try to feel the full impact of what this child has been through and how he or she feels as a result."

The interview was with a girl named Sheri Summers—"a very brave, bright 10-year-old." Her painful terminal illness was described in detail, and she talked about how she would love to get the services of the Quality Life Foundation. Subjects were then asked whether they wanted to fill out a special request to move Sheri up the waiting list. It was made clear that if this request were granted it would mean that other children higher up in priority would have to wait longer to get care.

The effect was strong. Three-quarters of the subjects in the high-empathy condition wanted to move her up, as compared to one-third in the low-empathy condition. Empathy's effects, then, weren't in the direction of increasing an interest in justice. Rather, they increased special concern for the target of the empathy, despite the cost to others.

This sort of effect takes us back to the metaphor of empathy as a spotlight. The metaphor captures a feature of empathy that its fans are quick to emphasize—how it makes visible the suffering of others, makes their troubles real, salient, and concrete. From the gloom, something is seen. Someone who believes we wouldn't help if it weren't for empathy might see its spotlight nature as its finest aspect.

But the metaphor also illustrates empathy's weaknesses. A spotlight picks out a certain space to illuminate and leaves the rest in darkness; its focus is narrow. What you see depends on where you choose to point the spotlight, so its focus is vulnerable to your biases.

Empathy is not the only facet of our moral lives that has a spotlight nature. Emotions such as anger, guilt, shame, and gratitude are similar. But not all psychological processes are limited in this way. We can engage in reasoning, including moral reasoning, that is more abstract. We can make decisions based on considerations of costs and benefits or through appealing to general principles. Presumably this is what the people who chose not to move Sheri Summers up the list were doing—they weren't zooming in on her, but rather taking a more distanced perspective. Now one might worry that this less emotional perspective is too cold and impersonal— maybe the right metaphor for this type of impartial reasoning is the ugly illumination of a fluorescent light. We'll get to that. My point here is just that the limitations of empathy are not inevitable.

Because of its spotlight properties, reliance on empathy can lead to perverse consequences, consequences that no rational person would endorse. You can see this in some fascinating psychological experiments.

In one study, subjects were given $10 and then told that they had the opportunity to give as much as they wanted to another individual who had nothing. All of this was anonymous; the other individual was just identified by a number, which the subject drew at random. The twist was that some of the subjects drew the number and then decided how much to give, while other subjects decided how much to give and then drew the number. Weirdly, people who drew the number first gave *far* more—60 percent more—than those who decided first, presumably because the prior drawing of the number helped them to imagine a specific person without money, as opposed to just some abstract individual.

In another study by the same research team, people were asked to donate money to Habitat for Humanity to help build a home for a family. They were told either that "the family has been selected" or that "the family will be selected." This subtle variation again made a difference. The subjects in the first condition gave a lot more, presumably because of the shift between a concrete target (the specific individuals who had been selected) and a more abstract one (those that will be selected in the future, who could be any of a large number).

Other studies compare how we respond to the suffering of one versus the suffering of many. Psychologists asked some subjects how much money they would give to help develop a drug that would save the life of one child, and asked others how much they would give to save eight children. People would give roughly the same in both cases. But when a third group of subjects were told the child's name and shown her picture, the donations shot up— now there were greater donations to the one than to the eight.

All of these laboratory effects can be seen as manifestations of what's been called "the identifiable victim effect." Thomas

Schelling, writing forty years ago, put it like this: "Let a six-year-old girl with brown hair need thousands of dollars for an operation that will prolong her life until Christmas, and the post office will be swamped with nickels and dimes to save her. But let it be reported that without a sales tax the hospital facilities of Massachusetts will deteriorate and cause a barely perceptible increase in preventable deaths—not many will drop a tear or reach for their checkbooks."

This effect also illustrates something more general about our natural sentiments, which is that they are *innumerate*. If our concern is driven by thoughts of the suffering of specific individuals, then it sets up a perverse situation in which the suffering of one can matter more than the suffering of a thousand.

To get a sense of the innumerate nature of our feelings, imagine reading that two hundred people just died in an earthquake in a remote country. How do you feel? Now imagine that you just discovered that the actual number of deaths was two thousand. Do you now feel ten times worse? Do you feel *any* worse?

I doubt it. Indeed, one individual can matter more than a hundred because a single individual can evoke feelings in a way that a multitude cannot. Stalin has been quoted as saying, "One death is a tragedy; one million is a statistic." And Mother Teresa once said, "If I look at the mass, I will never act. If I look at the one, I will." To the extent that we can recognize that the numbers are significant when it comes to moral decisions, it's because of reason, not sentiments.

One problem with spotlights is their narrow focus. Another is that they only light up what you point them at. They are vulnerable to bias.

The neuroscience research that we talked about earlier provided many illustrations of empathy's bias. Brain areas that correspond to the experience of empathy are sensitive to whether someone is a friend or a foe, part of one's group or part of an opposing group. Empathy is sensitive to whether the person is pleasing to look at or disgusting, and much else.

Just as with the identifiable victim effect, we can see this bias in the real world. Think about some of the events that have captured the sentiments of Americans over the last many decades.

There are girls in wells. In 1949, Kathy Fiscus, a three-year-old girl, fell into a well in San Marino, California, and the entire nation was seized with concern. Four decades later, America was transfixed by the plight of Jessica McClure—Baby Jessica—the eighteen-month-old who fell into a narrow well in Texas in October 1987, triggering a fifty-five-hour rescue operation. "Everybody in America became godmothers and godfathers of Jessica while this was going on," President Reagan remarked.

Larger-scale events can also engage us, so long as we can find identifiable victims in the crowd. So we resonate to certain tragedies, disasters, and great crimes, such the tsunami of 2004, Hurricane Katrina the year after, Hurricane Irene in 2011, Hurricane Sandy in 2012, and, of course, the attack on the Twin Towers on September 11, 2001. Or the example that began this book, when twenty children and six adults were murdered in Sandy Hook Elementary School in Newtown, Connecticut, leading to widespread grief and an intense desire to help.

These are all serious cases. But why these and not others? It's surely not their significance in any objective sense. Paul Slovic discusses the immense focus on Natalee Holloway, an eighteen-year-old American student who went missing on vacation in

Aruba and was believed to have been abducted and murdered. He points out that when Holloway went missing, the story of her plight took up far more television time than the concurrent genocide in Darfur. He notes that each day more than ten times the number of people who died in Hurricane Katrina die because of preventable diseases, and more than thirteen times as many die from malnutrition.

Plainly, then, the salience of these cases doesn't reflect an assessment of the extent of suffering, of their global importance, or of the extent to which it's possible for us to help. Rather, it reflects our natural biases in who to care about. We are fascinated by the plight of young children, particularly those who look like us and come from our community. In general, we care most about people who are similar to us—in attitude, in language, in appearance—and we will always care most of all about events that pertain to us and people we love.

Adam Smith made this point in 1790, using a now famous example. He asked us to suppose that everyone in China was killed in an earthquake. Then he imagined how "a man of humanity in Europe" would react: "He would, I imagine, first of all, express very strongly his sorrow for the misfortune of that unhappy people, he would make many melancholy reflections upon the precariousness of human life, and the vanity of all the labours of man, which could thus be annihilated in a moment. . . . And when all this fine philosophy was over, when all these humane sentiments had been once fairly expressed, he would pursue his business or his pleasure, take his repose or his diversion, with the same ease and tranquility as if no such accident had happened."

Smith then makes a comparison to the emotional response

evoked by a more personal event: "The most frivolous disaster which could befall himself would occasion a more real disturbance. If he was to lose his little finger to-morrow, he would not sleep to-night; but, provided he never saw them, he would snore with the most profound security over the ruin of a hundred millions of his brethren."

To modify Smith's example somewhat, suppose it wasn't you who were going to lose your little finger tomorrow. Suppose it was the person you were closest to, your young child perhaps. I bet you wouldn't sleep tonight. It would affect you far more than hearing about the deaths of multitudes in a faraway land. Actually, and this is a hard thing to write, I usually get more upset if my Internet connection becomes slow and uncertain than when I read about some tragedy in a country I haven't heard of.

There are exceptions; we can sometimes be drawn in by such distant events. But this typically happens when we are presented with images and stories that make the suffering salient, that serve to trigger those emotions and sentiments that would normally be activated by more local concerns.

The question of precisely how writers, producers, and journalists elicit moral concern is a fascinating topic and deserves a book of its own. But we know that it happens—literature, movies, television shows, and the like really have drawn people's attention to the suffering of strangers. Harriet Beecher Stowe's 1852 book *Uncle Tom's Cabin*, the best-selling novel of the nineteenth century, played a significant role in changing Americans' attitudes toward slavery. Dickens's *Oliver Twist* prompted changes in the way children were treated in nineteenth-century Britain. The work of Aleksandr Solzhenitsyn introduced people to the horrors of the Soviet gulag. Movies such as *Schindler's*

List and *Hotel Rwanda* expanded our awareness of the plight of people (sometimes in the past, sometimes in other countries) who we would otherwise never have cared about.

The choice of which of these distant events to focus on is itself influenced by the intuitions of journalists and filmmakers and novelists about which ones are most significant and which will resonate with a popular audience. As a result, some issues that matter to many people are hardly focused on at all. Stories about the horrific conditions inside American prisons rarely capture people's interest because, although they touch the lives of millions, most people don't care about those millions. Many see prison rape, for instance, as either a joke or a satisfying proof that what goes around, comes around.

Our selectivity in who to care about makes a difference. About twenty years ago, Walter Isaacson expressed his frustration over the American public's focus on the crisis in Somalia and relative disregard of the (objectively greater) tragedy in the Sudan, when he plaintively asked: "Will the world end up rescuing Somalia while ignoring the Sudan mainly because the former proves more photogenic?"

Before Somalia, there was the famine in Biafra. The journalist Philip Gourevitch tells how Americans were moved by the television coverage of "[s]tick-limbed, balloon-bellied, ancient-eyed" children. He goes on to recount how the State Department was flooded with mail, as many as twenty-five thousand letters in one day. It got to where President Lyndon Johnson told his undersecretary of state, "Just get those nigger babies off my TV set."

While writing this book, I discovered that there is a field of study called "disaster theory." A lot of the work in this area explores self-interested motivations. In the United States, for instance, presidents are more likely to declare national disasters during election years, and battleground states get more donations than others; money allocated to address disasters is used as an inducement and a reward. Other research in this area illustrates the arbitrariness of what we focus on, the way our interests fail to coincide with any reasonable assessment of where help is needed the most or where people can do the most good. This is the sort of thing Isaacson was complaining about.

Now some cases are difficult. Perhaps it's not obvious that it was wrong to prioritize Somalia over the Sudan, say. But some cases aren't hard at all, such as when concerns about adorable creatures—like oil-drenched penguins or, in 2014, a dog with Ebola that cost the city of Dallas $27,000 to care for—sap money and interest that could be better used to save lives.

I am *not* arguing that all the biases I have been discussing reflect the workings of empathy. Some do. It's a lot easier to empathize with someone who is similar to you, or someone who has been kind to you in the past, or someone you love, and because of this, these are the individuals you are more likely to help. The same empathic biases that show up in neuroscience laboratories influence us in our day-to-day interactions.

But other biases have causes that go deeper than empathy. We are constituted to favor our friends and family over strangers, to care more about members of our own group than people from different, perhaps opposing, groups. This fact about human nature is inevitable given our evolutionary history. Any creature that didn't have special sentiments toward those that shared its genes and helped it in the past would get its ass kicked from a Darwinian perspective; it would falter relative to competitors with more parochial natures. This bias to favor those close to us is general—it influences who we readily empathize with, but it also influences who we like, who we tend to care for, who we will affiliate with, who we will punish, and so on. Its scope is far broader than empathy.

Other biases arise out of facts about the way attention works. New things interest us; we grow insensitive to the same old same old. Just as we can come to ignore the hum of a refrigerator, we become inured to problems that seem unrelenting, like the starvation of children in Africa—or homicide in the United States. Mass shootings get splashed onto television screens, newspaper headlines, and the Web; the major ones settle into our collective memory—Columbine, Virginia Tech, Aurora, Sandy Hook. The 99.9 percent of other homicides are, unless the victim is someone you know, mere background noise.

Such biases are separate from empathy. But the spotlight nature of empathy means that *it is vulnerable to them*. Empathy's narrow focus, specificity, and innumeracy mean that it's always going to be influenced by what captures our attention, by racial preferences, and so on. It's only when we escape from empathy and rely instead on the application of rules and principles or a calculation of costs and benefits that we can, to at least some extent, become fair and impartial.

Are these biases really such a problem? People who worry about them might bring up the zero-sum nature of kindness. Money and time are finite. Every cent that I send to Save the Whales doesn't go to Oxfam; every hour spent knocking on doors seeking funds for a local art museum isn't spent working to help the homeless.

But so what? Maybe we're not perfect. Suppose it's true that our motivations to help others are racist and parochial and otherwise biased. Still, this is better than nothing. Maybe empathy and similar sentiments steer our helping of others in the wrong way, but without them we wouldn't help others in the first place. After all, the zero-sum nature of kindness is only a valid concern if someone is going to give or volunteer in the first place. If one is going to do something good, and empathy motivates one to do something less good, then empathy is to blame. But if one *isn't* going to do something good, and empathy motivates one to do it, then empathy is a plus.

Maybe complaining about empathy is like this joke: A Jewish grandmother is walking with her grandson on the beach when a wave comes in and pulls the boy into the ocean. She falls on her knees and weeps. She prays to God, "Bring him back to me. Oh God, please save my boy. Oh God, I would do anything." She continues to beseech God, and then, suddenly, another wave throws the boy onto the beach. He runs into her arms and the grandmother hugs him close. Then she looks up and says, with some annoyance (you've got to do the voice here): *"He was wearing a hat."*

Yes, God could have returned the hat, but really, is it appropriate to complain?

Keeping this in mind, consider Peter Singer's example of the misdirected focus that our sentiments generate. Miles Scott, a five-year-old with leukemia, was helped by the Make-A-Wish Foundation to spend the day as a superhero—Batkid. He drove through the city of San Francisco in a Batmobile with an actor dressed as Batman; he rescued a damsel in distress; he captured the Riddler; and he then received the keys of the city from the major of San Francisco, all while thousands of people cheered him on.

Singer admits that this gives him a warm glow. But then he asks about its price. The Make-A-Wish foundation says that the average cost for making a wish come true is $7,500. The Batkid scenario certainly cost more, but we can stick with this as a conservative estimate. Singer tells us that if this same money were used to provide bed nets in areas with malaria, it could save the lives of three children. And then he goes on: "It's obvious, isn't it, that saving a child's life is better than fulfilling a child's wish to be Batkid? If Miles's parents had been offered that choice— Batkid for a day or a complete cure for their son's leukemia— they surely would have chosen the cure. When more than one child's life can be saved, the choice is even clearer. Why then do so many people give to Make-A-Wish, when they could do more good by donating to the Against Malaria Foundation, which is a highly effective provider of bed nets to families in malaria-prone regions?"

Nobody would deny that it's better to save three children's lives than to give a single child a wonderful day. But one might object to Singer that this isn't the choice that people usually make. If people didn't donate the money to give the child his wish, it wouldn't have gone to save other children from malaria. It would have been used in ways that do even less good: a nicer car, a better vacation, some renovations to the kitchen. Good utilitarian that he is, Singer must appreciate that if those are the alternatives, it's better for the money to go to Batkid.

So I don't see the zero-sum argument as the biggest problem with the use of empathy to make decisions regarding charity. My worry is different.

It turns out that the kindness motivated by empathy often has bad effects. It can make the world worse. I'm not interested here in weird cases that a philosopher might think up, such as the example in the first chapter where someone saves a child from drowning and it turns out to be Hitler. Regardless of how we make our moral choices, we'll sometimes get things wrong. I am thinking of actual examples where, in sadly predictable ways, empathy leads to actions that have bad effects.

To see how this might happen, consider first a very different domain from charity. Think about parenting. A parent who lives too much in the head of his or her child will be overly protective and overly concerned, fearful, and uncertain, unable to exert any sort of discipline and control. Good parenting involves coping with the short-term suffering of your child—actually, sometimes *causing* the short-term suffering of your child. It involves denying children what they want—no, you can't eat cake for dinner/get a tattoo/go to a party on a school night. It involves imposing some degree of discipline, which almost by definition makes children's lives more unpleasant in the here and now. Empathy gets in the way of that, greedily focusing on the short-term buzz of increasing your children's happiness right now at the possible expense of what's actually good for them. It's sometimes said that the problem with parenting is overriding your own selfish concerns. But it turns out that another problem is overriding your *empathic* concerns: the strong desire to alleviate the immediate suffering of those around you.

Returning to the domain of charity, Singer points out that

many people are "warm glow" givers. They give small amounts to multiple charities, motivated to spread their money across many causes because each one gives a distinctive little jolt of pleasure, like plucking small treats from a bountiful table of desserts. But small donations can actually *harm* the charities, since the cost of processing a donation can be greater than the donation itself. Also, though Singer doesn't mention this, charities often follow up with donors, which is expensive for them, particularly if they send physical mail. If you want to harm some organization that supports a cause you object to, one mischievous way to do so is to send them a $5 donation.

As a far more serious issue, consider Western aid to developing nations. It turns out that there is considerable debate over how much of such aid actually helps and a growing consensus that a lot of it has a negative effect. Many worry that the clearly kindhearted intervention of affluent Westerners has made life worse for millions of people.

This might seem weird—what could be wrong about sending food to the hungry, giving medical aid to the ill, and so on? Part of the problem is that foreign aid decreases the incentives for long-term economic and social development in the areas that would most benefit from such development. Food aid can put local farmers and markets out of business. (These are the same sorts of concerns that arise domestically when people object to both welfare programs and corporate bailouts—the money might make things better at the moment, helping people keep their jobs, but it can have negative downstream consequences.) Then there is the concern that food aid and medical care for combatants, including those involved in genocide, can actually end up killing more people than it saves.

Also, the world contains unscrupulous people who exploit others, so empathy can be strategically triggered for bad ends. Consider orphanages. The feelings that many have for needy children motivate other individuals to establish a steady supply. Most children in Cambodia's orphanages, for instance, have at least one parent: Orphanages will pay or coerce poor parents to give up their children. A writer for the *New York Times* sums up the problem in a way that is consistent with the theme of this chapter: "The empathy of foreigners—who not only deliver contributions, but also sometimes open their own institutions— helped create a glut of orphanages. . . . Although some of the orphanages are clean and well-managed, many are decrepit and, according to the United Nations, leave children susceptible to sexual abuse. . . . 'Pity is a most dangerous emotion,' said Ou Virak, the founder of a human rights organization in Phnom Penh. 'Cambodia needs to get out of the beggar mentality. And foreigners need to stop reacting to pure emotion.'"

Or consider child beggars in the developing world. The sight of an emaciated child is shocking to a well-fed Westerner, and it's hard for a good person to resist helping out. And yet the act of doing so ends up supporting criminal organizations that enslave and often maim tens of thousands of children. By giving, you make the world worse. Actions that appear to help individuals in the short term can have terrible consequences for many more.

A discussion of unintended consequences might lead some to the conclusion that we shouldn't bother to help at all. This is *not* my argument. Many charities do wonderful work; kindness and hard work and charitable donations often make the world a better place in precisely the ways they are intended to. It's good to give blood, to provide bed nets to stop the spread of malaria, to read to the blind, and so on. Not everything is an O. Henry story with a dark twist at the end. Sometimes an obsessive concern with unintended consequences is just an excuse for selfishness and apathy.

But doing actual good, instead of doing what feels good, requires dealing with complex issues and being mindful of exploitation from competing, sometimes malicious and greedy, interests. To do so, you need to step back and not fall into empathy traps. The conclusion is not that one shouldn't give, but rather that one should give intelligently, with an eye toward consequences.

But, *still*, even if the spotlight nature of empathy sometime leads us astray, you might worry that if we gave up on empathy, we wouldn't do anything. We wouldn't care about anyone or anything besides ourselves, and the world would go to hell.

I think this view reflects an impoverished moral imagination, a failure to recognize the other forces that can give us empathy's benefits without all of its costs. We've already discussed many examples from everyday life where good acts—from saving a girl from drowning to donating a kidney—were not motivated by empathy. There are all sorts of motivations for good action. These include a diffuse concern or compassion, something that I'll return to in the next chapter. There are concerns about reputation, feelings of anger, pride, and guilt, and a commitment to religious and secular belief systems. We're too quick to credit empathy for what's right in the world.

To add another example to the mix, when I was a child I noticed that my father would sit at the kitchen table on some evenings and write out checks to the various charitable appeals that came in. He didn't empathically engage with the suffering that the appeals described—he barely read them. But when I asked him about it, he said he felt he had a general duty to help those less fortunate than himself. As I said, such indiscriminate giving has its risks, but it does illustrate, yet again, that if you step back and look at the good things that you and others do, you'll see that there is much more going on than the distorted and short-sighted force of empathy.

I have argued that being a good person involves some combination of caring for others—wanting to alleviate suffering and make the world a better place—and a rational assessment of how best to do so. It turns out that there is a project that focuses on exactly that, called "Effective Altruism," or EA. The Effective Altruists define themselves as: "a growing social movement that combines both the heart and the head." It's a good motto. The heart is needed to motivate you to do good; the head is the smarts to figure out how best to make that goodness happen.

This does not come easily. Zell Kravinsky, who donated his kidney to a stranger, said that people find this unusual only because "they don't understand math." But this isn't quite right— the real problem is that often people *don't care about math.*

But they can be persuaded to. People can be encouraged to think rationally about policy issues. Despite some skeptical claims to the contrary, people often wish to do the right thing, not merely what feels good. There are many who use resources such as givewell.org to monitor the efficacy of charities and determine which make the most difference. As Jennifer Rubenstein put it, this focus on empirically informed decisions championed by movements like EA makes it "far superior to charity appeals based on identifiable victims, charismatic megafauna (e.g., polar bears), charismatic mega-stars (e.g., Bono), oversimplified villains (e.g., Joseph Kony), and dramatic images of disaster."

Not everyone is a fan of Effective Altruism. When Peter Singer defended these ideas in a recent article in the *Boston Review*, several scholars and activists were asked to comment, and many were critical. Some accepted Singer's premise that we should focus on maximizing the positive consequences of our actions but objected to his specifics. It was argued that more good would be done if people put less energy into personal charitable donations and focused instead on lobbying for broad policy changes such as opposing arms trades or protectionist tariffs. Others argued that the most efficacious interventions are made by corporations, not individuals. And there were worries about unintended consequences, such as the concern that focusing on individual giving might erode support for large-scale responses by institutions like the U.S. government.

Singer's response to these sorts of critiques was measured, agreeing with some points, pushing back on others, and generally adopting the position that these are empirical questions to be decided on a case-by-case basis. I would add myself, following an argument by Scott Alexander, that one consideration in favor of Effective Altruism as it's currently carried out is its epistemic humility. Stopping the spread of malaria through bed nets might not be the ultimately best long-term solution for Third World problems, but most likely it does some good. In contrast, the outcome of broader political interventions is considerably less certain, and if the Effective Altruism movement went in that direction it would be indistinguishable from other political movements, and its unique contribution would be lost.

Expanding on this point, Alexander makes a distinction between "man versus nature" problems and "man versus man" problems. Healing the sick is an example of "man versus nature," and this is the sort of thing that effective altruists now focus on. Fighting global capitalism is "man versus man." This has the potential for long-lasting change for the better, but the outcome is less certain. After all, many people are in favor of global capitalism, and many honestly believe that the spread of market economies is what will make the world a better place.

All of this in the end comes down to empirical questions over what actions have the best overall benefit. What's more interesting to me as a psychologist is a different type of reaction that the EA proposal has evoked. Larissa MacFarquhar notes that to many—though perhaps not her—"it is disturbing to act upon people at such a distance that they become abstractions, even if the consequences are better"; she calls this "the drone program of altruism." Paul Brest complains about Effective Altruism's "sanctimonious attitude." Catherine Tumber discusses Singer's example of Matt Wage, a young man who went to Wall Street to make money so that he could give to the starving poor. She states that Wage's work actually "furthers the suffering of global have-nots" and that it degrades him as well—"it reflects a form of profound alienation."

Singer has less patience for these responses, and is particularly annoyed at Tumber's insistence that the money donated by Wage isn't doing any good for others (he asks how she knows this) and her more general objection to quantifying the amount of good that one can do. Singer says that her view "implies that she would be willing to support a charity that, say, will prevent blindness in a small number of people even when the same resources donated to a different charity would prevent blindness in many more people." He concludes, "It is hard to know what to say about such a preference."

I share Singer's reaction. A few years ago I was on a radio program talking about the last book I wrote—on the origins of morality in children—and got into a discussion with a pastor about how we deal with strangers, using the example of child beggars in the developing world. I tentatively raised the concern, which I had recently read about, that giving to these beggars makes things worse, causing more suffering, and suggested we should stop doing it; we should use our money in better ways.

Her response surprised me. She didn't challenge me on the facts; what she said was that she *liked* giving to beggars. She said that handing over food or money to a child, seeing the child's satisfaction, made her feel good. It's an important human contact, she told me, not the sort of thing you can ever get by typing your credit card number into oxfam.org.

I said nothing at the time, being both nonconfrontational and occasionally slow-witted. But if I could answer now, I would say that it depends on what you want. If you want the pleasure of personal contact, go ahead and give something to the child, perhaps feeling a little buzz when your hands touch, a warmness that sits with you as you walk back to your hotel. If you actually want to make people's lives better, do something different.

Singer's critics are right to point out that people have priorities other than health and security. People want to be treated with respect, for instance, and they often want to play an active role in their own improvement. And when we think about costs and benefits, we should also consider the lives of affluent Westerners. To the extent that Tumber is right and Matt Wage's life is diminished through devoting his career to helping the poor, that's something that needs to be tossed into the mix. I appreciate as well that there's something cold and dissatisfying about charity at a distance. Someone I know well, an affluent professor, spent a period of her life regularly working as a volunteer in a New Haven soup kitchen, even though she knew that she would do far more good by writing a check. She wanted the contact. I don't dismiss this. When it comes to adding up the costs and benefits of an action, surely the satisfaction of a Yale professor has some weight.

But I'd give it a lot less weight than the needs of those who are actually suffering. If a child is starving, it doesn't really matter whether the food is delivered by a smiling aid worker who hands it over and then gives the kid a hug, or dropped from the sky by a buzzing drone. The niceties of personal contact are far less important than actually saving lives.

One of the most thoughtful analyses of the weaknesses of empathy comes from Elaine Scarry, in a brief article called "The Difficulty of Imagining Other People." Her approach is different from mine but, I think, nicely complementary.

Scarry starts in a pro-empathy mode, noting that our treatment of other people is shaped by how we imagine their lives. She goes so far as to say that *"the human capacity to injure other people is very great precisely because our capacity to imagine other people is very small"* (her italics). She then asks how members of a society can be motivated to act better to strangers and foreigners, and she considers an empathic solution—"a framework of cosmopolitan largesse that relies on the population to spontaneously and generously 'imagine' other persons and to do so on a day-to-day basis."

This solution has many fans in international policy circles and is supported as well by philosophers such as Martha Nussbaum, who has elaborated on the importance of empathy in our treatment of others, including those in faraway lands. Some novelists are drawn by this view, seeing one of the benefits of fiction as the expansion of the moral imagination. George Eliot argued in 1856 that kindness to others requires some sort of emotive push: "Appeals founded on generalizations and statistics require a sympathy readymade, a moral sentiment already in activity," and suggested that this could arise through fiction and other arts. She concluded that "a picture of human life such as a great artist can give, surprises even the trivial and the selfish into that attention to what is apart from themselves, which may be called the raw material of moral Sentiment."

Scarry is unconvinced. She worries that our imaginings of the lives of others don't provide enough motivation to elicit kindness. Her skepticism isn't rooted in the sort of experimental work that we've been talking about here. Instead, she draws on everyday intuition and experience. She points out that it's hard to vividly imagine even a close friend with the same intensity that one experiences oneself. To do this for large numbers of strangers, such as (her examples) the Turks residing in Germany, the undocumented immigrants in the United States, the multitudes of Iraqi soldiers and citizens killed in bombing raids, is just impossible.

These observations bring us back to a complaint I've made before—empathy is innumerate and biased. Hearing that my child has been mildly harmed is far more moving for me than hearing about the horrific death of thousands of strangers. This might be a fine attitude for a father—we'll return to that question at the end of the next chapter—but it's a poor attitude for a policy maker and a poor moral guide to our treatment of strangers.

A common response here is that we should try harder to feel for others. Now, this might be a worthy demand when it comes to a specific individual, perhaps someone whose suffering I am ignoring or even causing. But it's bad advice when many people are involved, including strangers. We are not psychologically constituted to feel toward a stranger as we feel toward someone we love. We are not capable of feeling a million times worse about the suffering of a million than about the suffering of one. Our gut feelings provide the wrong currency through which to evaluate our own moral actions.

Scarry's proposed alternative is similar to mine. She notes that someone who relies on empathy will focus on individuals with the goal of making their lives *weighty,* of making their joy and suffering and experience matter as much as one's own. This sounds noble, but we are not good at it. A prosperous American, for instance, cannot make the life of a starving African child as weighty as the lives of his or her own children. And nobody can evaluate the consequences of something like global warming or a future war by making individual lives more weighty, because there are no specific lives to do this with, just abstract generalities.

Scarry suggests that we do the opposite. Don't try to establish equality and justice by raising others up to the level of those you love. Don't try to make them more weighty. Rather, *make yourself less weighty*. Bring everyone to the same level by diminishing yourself. Put yourself, and those you love, on the level of strangers.

We see this sort of advice spelled out by Bertrand Russell, who says that when we read the newspaper, we ought to substitute the names of countries, including our own, to get a more fair sense of what's going on. Take "Israel" and replace it with "Bolivia," replace "United States" with "Argentina," and so on. (Perhaps even better would be to use arbitrary symbols: X, Y, and Z.) This is an excellent way to remove bias. As Scarry puts it, "The veil of ignorance fosters equality not by giving the millions of other people an imaginative weight equal to one's own—a staggering mental labor—but by the much more efficient strategy of simply erasing for the moment one's own dense array of attributes."

Scarry's idea, then, is to depersonalize things, to bring everyone down rather than bringing everyone up. I admit that this sounds cold. It might also seem like aiming too low. It's like Louis CK's advice about how to have exactly the body you want: "You just have to want a shitty body. That's all it is. You have to want your own shitty, ugly, disgusting body." But since we can't empathize with everyone to the same extent, this may well be the best procedure we will ever have.

And such depersonalization is already at the core of wise policies. When we want to make fair and unbiased decisions about who to hire or who to give an award to, we don't give everyone equal "imaginative weight," fully appreciating the special circumstances and humanity of each individual. No, we instead reduce our candidates to X, Y, and Z, designing procedures, such as blind reviewing and blind auditions, to prevent judges from being biased, consciously or unconsciously, by a candidate's sex, race, appearance—or anything other than what should be under evaluation. Alternatively, we can establish quota systems and diversity requirements to ensure sufficient representation by certain groups. These are conflicting solutions, grounded in different political visions, but they are both attempts to depersonalize the process and circumvent our natural preferences and biases.

As an example, suppose you are on a panel choosing who gets a prestigious award, and a nomination comes in for your daughter. Do you try to expand your feelings toward all the other candidates so that you love everyone equally and can now be fair? Hardly. Instead, you withdraw from that decision, handing it to over to judges who can see your daughter as yet another stranger, on a par with the other applicants.

It's easy to misunderstand what these sorts of appeals to impartiality are really about. In a discussion of an article where I endorse a similar proposal, Simon Baron-Cohen presents a dark vision of a world without empathic decision makers: "If we leave empathy out of our decision making we are in danger of doing what the Nazis did: designing a perfectly rational system such as the Final Solution, with trains taking Jews from all over Europe to the concentration camps and their perfectly designed system of gas chambers and ovens. It all made sense from a Nazi perspective, if the aim was to eradicate anyone with impure blood. All that was missing was empathy for the Jewish victims."

He goes on to describe what he sees as the outcome of cost-benefit decision-making: "Or consider how the Nazis designed a euthanasia program to systematically eradicate people with learning difficulties. The cost-benefit argument was irrefutable:

Euthanasia removes 'diseased genes' from the population and saves money, since the cost of supporting a person with life-long learning difficulties was high. What enabled these legal decisions—what allowed lawmakers to believe they were being moral—was the absence of empathy for people with learning difficulties."

For Baron-Cohen, the costs and benefits are *financial* costs and benefits. This is why he concludes that, from a rational point of view, the cost-benefit argument for Nazi euthanasia of those with learning difficulties is "irrefutable," as it saves the government money.

Now this sort of cost-benefit calculation would truly be grotesque. But it's not what I am proposing (or what anyone is proposing, as far as I know). Rather, my alternative to empathy includes compassion for others, so any rational decision-making process would take happiness and thriving and suffering into account. To put it in Baron-Cohen's terms, if we did a cost-benefit analysis, the mass murder of the learning disabled would be an intolerable cost.

This might be an off-putting way to frame things, and Baron-Cohen is not alone in scorning those who engage in rational deliberations. But I am a proponent of that approach, and this is going to lead me to what might be the most controversial part of this book.

I am going to say something nice about economists. This doesn't come easy to me. As a professor, I can tell you that they are hardly the most popular individuals in a university, with their ridiculous salaries, fine suits, and repeated failures to warn us when the economy is about to go belly up. But their application of cold economic reasoning sometimes puts them on the side of the angels, as they work to be professionally immune to the sorts of prejudices and biases that most people are subject to.

For instance, most economists believe in the merits of free trade, and this is in large part because, unlike politicians and many citizens, they refuse to see any principled difference between the lives of people in our country and the lives of people in others. An American president who claimed that we shouldn't fight to keep jobs in America—after all, Mexican families are just as important as families in the United States— wouldn't be president much longer. But economists dismiss this as sheer bias that makes the world worse.

Or consider why economics is sometimes called "the dismal science." It's a derogatory description thought up by Thomas Carlyle in the 1800s, coined to draw a contrast with the "gay science" of music and poetry: "Not a 'gay science,' I should say, like some we have heard of; no, a dreary, desolate and, indeed, quite abject and distressing one; what we might call, by way of eminence, the *dismal science*."

Carlyle has a specific issue in mind, a case where he wanted to ridicule economists for objecting to something that was the subject of considerable feeling and heart, something that Carlyle had defended with great emotion.

What was this issue that the economists were being so negative about? Slavery. Carlyle was upset because the economists were *against slavery*. He argued for the reintroduction of slavery in the West Indies and was annoyed that the economists railed against it. Think about this when you're tempted to scorn economists and the cool approach they take to human affairs, and when you hear people equating strong feelings with goodness and cold reason with nastiness. In the real world, as we've seen, the truth is usually the opposite.

The Politics of Empathy

When arguing against empathy, I'm often challenged about my politics. Am I pursuing some sort of conservative agenda here? Is this intended as a thumb in the eye to liberals and progressives?

It's a natural question to ask. Many people think of empathy as associated with a cluster of views that are liberal, left-wing, and progressive. In the United States, at least, these include being in favor of gay marriage, stricter gun control, increased access to abortion, more open borders, and government programs such as universal health care. Those who hold these views are often seen as particularly empathic.

To say that liberals are more empathic than conservatives can mean two subtly different things. One can be talking about the political philosophies themselves. George Lakoff, an enthusiastic supporter of liberal causes, puts it in its strongest terms: "Behind every progressive policy lies a single moral value: empathy." Alternatively, one could be talking about individual liberals and individual conservatives. Perhaps more empathic people tend to adopt more liberal views than conservative views;

or maybe being exposed to liberal ideas makes one more empathic, while exposure to conservative views makes one less.

The claim about positions and the claim about individuals are logically distinct—it's possible, for instance, that liberals are more empathic, but the philosophy of liberalism itself doesn't have any special association with empathy—but they are obviously related. It would make sense that more empathic people would go for the more empathic political vision and that less empathic people would be drawn to the less empathic political philosophy.

In any case, if it's true that liberal policies are rooted in empathy *and* if I'm right that empathy is a poor moral guide, then what you are looking at in this book is an attack on the left. This would certainly be an interesting position to take.

But it is not my argument. It turns out that there is some association between empathy and politics, along the directions that you'd expect. But this association is not as strong as people believe it is. There are conservative positions that are deeply grounded in empathy and liberal positions that are not. Being against empathy won't tell you what to think about gun control, taxation, health care, and the like; it won't tell you who to vote for, or what your general political philosophy should be.

For better or worse, then, my attack on empathy is nonpartisan. Or to put it more positively, individuals of all political orientations—liberal, conservative, libertarian, hard right, hard left, all of us—can join hands and work together in the fight against empathy.

To talk about this issue at all, we need to think about what it means to be liberal/progressive/left-wing or conservative/right-wing. These words have changed meanings over time, and political language is itself the focus of intense political debate. There are those on the far left who hate "liberals" and "liberalism," and most of all "neoliberalism," with great passion. Many views associated with "conservatism" are not, in any literal sense, conservative; they are actually radical, such as dismantling government programs that have been in place for a long time. Libertarians, who are not categorized as liberal in the modern political sphere—because of their enthusiasm for free market policies and their disdain for certain social programs—will often insist that they are the real liberals, defenders of the policies of the founders of liberalism such as John Locke and John Stuart Mill.

These are intricate and complex issues, and I plan to duck all of them. In what follows, I'm going to use phrases like left/liberal/progressive and right/conservative in the usual way that nonacademic Americans and Europeans do. I do so because this corresponds to what people are talking about when they say that liberals are more empathic than conservatives. That is, when people associate liberals with empathy, they think of liberals in the usual way that they are talked about in everyday discourse—as those who want greater legal protection for sexual and ethnic minorities, who worry about the proliferation of guns, who favor legal access to abortion, who support diversity programs in universities, who support universal health care, and so on.

I should add that, at least in the United States, people aren't being irrational in carving up the political world in this way. It turns out that the commonsense categories of liberal and conservative do a surprisingly good job of capturing the cluster of views that people possess. It didn't have to work that way; specific political views could have turned out to be independent of each other—it could have been, say, that views on gun control have nothing to do with views on gay marriage, in the same way that your favorite pizza topping is unrelated to whether you like the *Mission Impossible* movies. But there are by now count-less studies looking at political orientation and asking people whether they are liberal or conservative, and it turns out that this sort of crude assessment works just fine at predicting all sorts of specific views. For instance, one study asked people about the following five issues:

- Stricter gun control laws in the United States
- Universal health care
- Raising income taxes for persons in the highest income-tax bracket
- Affirmative action for minorities
- Stricter carbon emission standards to reduce global warming

If you are American or European, you'll have strong intu-itions about which positions on these issues correspond to the liberal side and which to the conservative side, and you'll be right. Moreover, these views hang together; people who approve one of them tend to approve the others; people who oppose one of them tend to oppose the others. These broader patterns of approval and disapproval correspond to where people place themselves on a left-right scale, liberal (or progressive) versus conservative. If you want to know people's views, then, a per-fectly good question is "Are you liberal or conservative?"

Indeed, some believe that a political continuum from left to right might be universal. John Stuart Mill pointed out that political systems have "a party of order or stability and a party of progress or reform." Ralph Waldo Emerson wrote that "the two parties which divide the state, the party of conservatism and that of innovation, are very old, and have disputed the possession of the world ever since it was made," and he went on to conclude that such "irreconcilable antagonism must have a correspondent depth of seat in the human condition."

This antagonism is stronger with social issues. Our political natures seem to manifest themselves most clearly with, as one set of scholars put it, "matters of reproduction, relations with out-groups, suitable punishment for in-group miscreants, and traditional/innovative lifestyles." Less intimate issues, such as free trade or deregulation of banks, are less predictable and aren't as reliably related to one's broader political orientation.

Not surprisingly, there is a rough correlation in the United States between political orientation and membership in the major political parties; those who see themselves as liberals tend to vote Democratic and those who see themselves as conservatives tend to vote Republican. But the relationship is far from perfect: On a scale from 0 to 1, the correlation between political views and party membership is about 0.5 to 0.6.

The relationship is imperfect in part because party membership is determined by factors other than ideology, particularly at the more local level, where the issues aren't gay rights or abortion but snow emergencies and property taxes. Also, the two main political parties are ideologically heterogeneous. In the 2012 U.S. presidential election, for instance, the contenders in the Republican primary included Rick Santorum, who was concerned about sexual purity, a central role of religion in public life, and a strong military—the perfect embodiment of a socially conservative worldview—and the libertarian Ron Paul, whose philosophy demands maximum personal freedom in everyday life and a far less aggressive foreign policy.

So are liberals more empathic? It seems so. It is probably no accident that Barack Obama, who talks more about empathy than any president in history, is a Democrat. It was his Democratic predecessor, Bill Clinton, who famously said to Americans, "I feel your pain." Other prominent Democrats use the language of empathy with some fluidity. In the wake of the choke hold death of Eric Garner at the hands of New York City police officers, Hilary Clinton called for changing police tactics, and then said: "The most important thing each of us can do is to try even harder to see the world through our neighbors' eyes. . . . To imagine what it is like to walk in their shoes, to share their pain and their hopes and their dreams."

Many see this way of thinking as reflecting something central in the liberal worldview—increased empathy is what ties together the policies that liberals endorse. One analysis, by psychologists who study the relationship between politics and empathy, goes as follows: "To the extent that citizens identify with the distresses of others, they will prefer to assuage the distress that they witness. In the political realm, such actions would likely entail the invocation of government power on behalf of the perceived victims. Hence, 'bleeding hearts,' we hypothesize, would prefer liberal policy solutions to remedy problems encountered by distressed, generalized others."

To the extent, then, that one political party is saying that you should help people in need by loosening immigration restrictions or raising the minimum wage, it makes sense that the people who belong to that group are motivated by empathy—a lot more so than those who oppose these views. To see what a different sort of rhetoric looks like, Obama's opponent during the 2012 election, the Republican Mitt Romney, was ridiculed for saying, "I like being able to fire people who provide services to me." Now Romney was making a legitimate point about the workings of an economic system that he favors and the way he believes that it ultimately makes everyone better off, but it is an almost comically *un*empathic position to take.

Many liberals would sum this all up by saying that they are the caring ones, while conservatives are vindictive, cruel, punitive, and unfeeling. Liberals want to increase the minimum wage because they care about poor people; conservatives don't. Liberals want stricter gun laws because they worry about the victims of gun violence; conservatives don't. Liberals favor abortion rights because they care about women, while conservatives want to restrict women's freedom. This is George Lakoff's analysis of the antiabortion position: Conservatives think of society as an authoritarian traditional family, and when it comes to abortion, "The very idea that a women can make such a decision—a decision over her own reproduction, over her own body, and over a man's progeny—contradicts and represents a threat to the idea of a strict father morality."

This is conservatism as seen by its worst enemies. But conservatives themselves may resonate to being less empathic. After all, they accuse liberals of being softheaded and emotional— "bleeding hearts" and "tree huggers" are hardly compliments. They might approvingly repeat the line often attributed to Winston Churchill: "If you're not a liberal at twenty you have no heart; if you're not a conservative at forty you have no brain." Conservatives might argue for the importance of nonempathic moral values, such as greater emphasis on tradition, including religious tradition, and greater emphasis on individual rights and freedoms.

Conservatives also tend to have a certain skepticism about the extent of human kindness, particularly toward those who are not family and friends, and they worry as well about the unreliability and corruptibility of state institutions. While liberals advocate for government programs that they believe make the world a better place—universal health care, say, or universal early education programs such as Head Start—conservatives worry that these never work out as planned.

A different analysis of the liberal-conservative contrast is proposed by Jonathan Haidt, based on his theory that humans possess a set of distinct moral foundations—including those concerning care, fairness, loyalty, authority, and sanctity. These are evolved universals, but they admit of variation, and research by Haidt and his colleagues suggests that liberals emphasize care and fairness over the others, while conservatives care about all these foundations more or less equally. This is why, according to Haidt, conservatives care more than liberals do about respect for the national flag (as this is associated with loyalty), children's obedience toward parents (authority), and chastity (sanctity). And again this perspective has conservatives drawing upon nonempathic values more so than liberals.

Finally, there is research on the actual mind-sets of liberals and conservatives. One study, using online survey methods, tested about seven thousand people, asking them for their political affiliations and then testing them on two standard empathy measures: Davis's "empathic concern" scale and Baron-Cohen's "empathizer" scale. I complained about both of these scales in an earlier chapter, pointing out, among other things, that they measure traits other than empathy and that they are vulnerable to self-report and self-perception biases (they measure what you think you are like, not necessarily what you are actually like). But still, they probably do capture *something* having to do with empathy, and exactly as one would predict, self-defined liberals are significantly more empathic than self-defined conservatives on both scales. These are not huge differences, but they are real ones.

Finally, if it turns out that being liberal is more attractive to empathic people, this could help make sense of the fact that women are statistically more likely to be liberal than men, since women tend to be somewhat more empathic than men. The authors of one study that looked at empathy, gender, and political orientation conclude that if males were as empathic as females, the gender gap in politics would almost entirely disappear.

So there is something to the idea that a liberal worldview is more empathic than a conservative one. But this connection between political ideology and empathy is not as strong as it might first appear.

For one thing, even the stereotypes are more nuanced. Some prominent liberal politicians — Michael Dukakis comes to mind, perhaps Al Gore as well — are seen as, and present themselves as, rational technocrats, careful problem solvers. And some more conservative politicians — such as Ronald Reagan — are remarkably good at presenting themselves as empathically connected to others.

More to the point, it is too crude to associate liberal policies with empathy. Consider that many policies associated with liberalism are also endorsed by libertarians, who are, by standard empathy measures, the least empathic individuals of all. Liberals and libertarians share common cause over issues such as gay marriage, the legalization of some drugs, and the militarization of the police. If such policies are grounded in empathy, it is mysterious why the least empathic people on earth would also endorse them.

In addition, certain conservative policies also draw upon empathic concerns for specific individuals. They just happen to be different individuals than those the liberals are empathizing with. So liberals in favor of open borders may try to evoke empathy for the suffering of refugees, while their conservative counterparts will talk about Americans who might lose their jobs. Liberals might empathize deeply with minorities who they feel are abused or threatened by the police, but conservatives empathize with police officers and with those owners of small businesses who have lost their livelihoods in riots sparked by protests against the police.

These figure/ground shifts in perspective, where there is a flip between who is the focus of concern, are endemic in political debate. Political debates typically involve a disagreement not over whether we should empathize, but over who we should empathize with.

Take gun control. Liberals often argue for gun control by focusing on the victims of gun violence. But conservatives point to those who have their guns taken away from them, now defenseless against the savagery of others. Smart politicians appreciate this symmetry. When Barack Obama was talking to the Denver

Police Academy, he recounted that, while campaigning in Iowa, Michelle Obama told him this: "You know, if I was living out on a farm in Iowa, I'd probably want a gun, too. When somebody just drives up into your driveway and you're not home, you don't know who these people are, you don't know how long it's going to take for the sheriffs to respond, I can see why you'd want some guns for protection."

Characteristically, Obama suggested that the solution to this clash of empathic concerns is yet more empathy. He went on to suggest that we "put each other in the other person's shoes," and that hunters and sportsmen should imagine what it's like to be a mother who has lost her son to a random act of violence, and vice versa.

Or take concerns about the use of torture by the CIA and the American military. It might seem that empathy can favor only one side of the debate there—concerns about the suffering of those who are tortured. But this is too simple. After the publication of the torture reports in late 2014, ex-vice-president Dick Cheney was asked to defend the United States' record on torture. Now you might imagine that his argument would involve abstract appeals to security and safety. And yet when asked to define torture, Cheney gave this example: "an American citizen on a cell phone making a last call to his four young daughters shortly before he burns to death in the upper levels of the Trade Center in New York City on 9/11." This is an empathic argument, defending torture by talking about the suffering of a single identifiable individual.

Or consider concerns about certain sorts of expression. Liberals worry about the offense caused by racist and sexist speech; conservatives worry about the offense caused by speech that belittles traditional values. Both liberals and conservatives object, for different reasons, to certain overt displays of sexuality, and they often find common cause in battling pornography. Both protest the ridicule of certain esteemed figures (different ones, of course) and can be quick to demand that people be fired, humiliated, or at the very least forced to apologize, when saying something offensive on social media.

It's this sort of thing that should make one worry about the role of empathy in our political lives. The problem isn't that all these concerns are mistaken. Even the most zealous defender of free speech believes in some restrictions: Most believe that it's legitimate to fire an elementary school teacher who teaches Nazi ideology, say, or to curtail someone from screaming racist epithets at people on the street. And some remarks on social media really do deserve a sharp response. But the problem is that empathy is always on the side of the censor. It is easy to feel the pain of the person who is upset by speech, and particularly easy to do so if the person is part of your community and is bothered by the same things you are. It seems mighty cold-blooded to tell someone who has been really hurt that they should just suck it up.

The case for free speech, in contrast, is pretty unempathic. There are many arguments for why we should be reluctant to restrict the speech of others, some of them drawing on consequentialist concerns (the world is better off in the long run if all ideas, even bad ones, get an airing), some of them based on conceptions of human freedom in which the right to self-expression is paramount. There is also an enlightened form of self-interest going on in a defense of free speech: You get the right to say what you want, and in return I get that right for myself. But none of these are particularly empathic considerations, and, here, as elsewhere, a reasonable public policy draws upon more general, and less biased, motivations.

Empathy also shows its nonpartisan nature in the legal context. Many liberals, including Obama, have argued for the need for empathic judges, and this is routinely scorned by conservatives as an attempt to bias the legal system in favor of liberal causes. But in a thoughtful discussion, Thomas Colby points out that conservative Supreme Court Justices are just as prone as liberal ones to raise empathic concerns. That is, even the most conservative justices, though they sometimes describe judicial decision-making as a mechanical process—like an umpire calling balls and strikes, as John Roberts put it—tacitly accept the importance of empathic considerations.

And sometimes not so tacitly. In his confirmation hearing, Clarence Thomas suggested that his unique contribution as a justice would be that he "can walk in the shoes of the people who are affected by what the Court does," while Samuel Alito, in his own hearing, noted that "When I get a case about discrimination, I have to think about people in my own family who suffered discrimination because of their ethnic background or because of religion or because of gender, and I do take that into account."

More relevantly, certain decisions made by conservative justices are plainly grounded in empathy. Colby gives the example of Alito's dissent in a free speech case involving protesting at military funerals by the Westboro Baptist Church, where Alito cited the "severe and lasting emotional injury" and the "acute emotional vulnerability" experienced by the families of the deceased. But the other justices were unanimous in their view that these protests, however reprehensible, were fully legal, and Colby speculates that Alito let his empathy motivate a decision that runs contrary to the law.

We've seen how conservatives can rely on empathy just as much as liberals. More than that, certain perspectives associated with liberal philosophies aren't that empathic at all.

The best example of this is climate change, something that progressives care more about than conservatives. Here, empathy favors doing nothing. If you do act, many identifiable victims— real people who we can feel empathy for—will be harmed by increased gas prices, business closures, increased taxes, and so on. The millions or billions of people who at some unspecified future date will suffer the consequences of our current inaction are, by contrast, pale statistical abstractions. When liberals argue that we should act, something other than empathy is involved.

We see, then, that there is no Party of Empathy. It's not that liberal policies are driven by empathy and conservative ones are not. A more realistic perspective is that a politics of empathy drives concerns about people in the here and now. This meshes well with some liberal causes and some conservative causes. In some cases, such as gun control, empathy pushes both ways; in others, such as free speech and climate change, it is mostly silent on one side.

There are worse things than caring about people in the here and now, of course. If you are in a position to make suffering go away, you should act, and sometimes worries about long-term effects are just rationalizations for apathy and self-interest. Still, the cost of a politics of empathy is massive. Governments' failures to enact prudent long-term policies are often attributed to the incentive system of democratic politics (which favors short-term fixes) and to the powerful influence of money. But the politics of empathy is also to blame. It is because of empathy that citizens of a country can be transfixed by a girl stuck in a well and largely indifferent to climate change. It is because of empathy that we often enact savage laws or enter into terrible wars; our feeling for the suffering of the few leads to disastrous consequences for the many.

A reasoned, even counterempathic analysis of moral obligation and likely consequences is a better guide to planning for the future than the gut wrench of empathy. This is not a partisan point; it's a sensible one.

CHAPTER 4

Intimacy

What are you looking for in a romantic partner? A team of psychologists once asked thousands of people from dozens of cultures about the qualities they wanted in a mate. The researchers were interested in sex differences, so they asked about traits like youth, chastity, power and wealth, and good looks—just those traits that one would expect to be relevant from an evolutionary psychology perspective. Some sex differences were found, mostly along the predicted directions (men cared more about youth; women about status), and commentators on the article argued about the precise nature of these differences and whether they reflect biological forces or cultural norms.

But what was largely ignored in all this was that men and women agreed on the number one factor when it comes to a mate. It wasn't age or looks or wealth. It was *kindness*.

For a lot of people, this means empathy. To my knowledge, nobody has yet done a study that specifically asks how people rank empathy when looking for a romantic partner, but I bet it would matter a lot. If you're looking for love and you're not an empathic person, I'd recommend that you keep this to yourself, at least on the first date. Common sense tells us that for all sorts of relationships—not just for friends and family but also for more professional relationships such as doctors and therapists, coaches, and teachers—the more empathy the better.

Now part of this is because the word *empathy* means, for many people, everything that is morally good—compassion, warmth, understanding, caring, and so on. But suppose we consider empathy in the more narrow sense I've been interested in throughout this book—the capacity for feeling what others feel. My sense is that many people would still say that more empathic people make better partners and friends. Are they wrong?

My arguments against empathy up to now have been mostly at the policy level. But intimate relationships are a different story, and I haven't yet given any reasons to question the value of empathy in the personal realm.

Perhaps there aren't any reasons to be had. After all, the factors that make empathy so problematic in the policy domain, such as how biased it is, might not be problems when things get more personal. In fact they may be advantages. Adam Smith talked about the moral importance of overriding the power of the passions, including empathy, and how important it is that we come to appreciate that "we are but one of the multitude, in no respect better than any other in it." But while this may be an excellent recipe for fair and impartial moral decision-making, I don't want my sons or my friends or my wife to see me as "one of the multitude"! Most of us, I presume, wish to be special in the eyes of those we love and who love us. For that, the spotlight nature of empathy seems just the ticket.

Consider also that empathy might have evolved in our species to facilitate one-on-one relationships, such as those between parents and young children. Empathy's failures would be expected to arise when it's extended to situations it hasn't been shaped for, in which we have to assess the consequences of our acts in a world filled with strangers. But intimate relationships are its bailiwick, so we should expect it to be most useful here.

In the first article I wrote on the topic, I made a case for this: "Where empathy really does matter is in our personal relationships. Nobody wants to live like Thomas Gradgrind—Charles Dickens's caricature utilitarian, who treats all interactions, including those with his children, in explicitly economic terms. Empathy is what makes us human; it's what makes us both subjects and objects of moral concern. Empathy betrays us only when we take it as a moral guide."

For reasons of space, my editor wanted to cut these sentences, but I insisted on keeping them because it was important to me at the time that readers not believe I'm against empathy altogether. This seemed like an extreme and somewhat weird view, not something I wanted to be associated with.

I'm no longer so certain. A careful look at empathy reveals a more complicated story. Here as always it's important to distinguish empathy from understanding. It's undeniably a good thing when the people in our lives understand us. And it's even more important to distinguish empathy from compassion, warmth, and kindness. Nobody could deny that we want the people in our lives to care about us.

But what if we zoom in on the capacity for empathy in the Adam Smith sense of feeling people's pain and pleasure, of experiencing the world as they experience it? How important is *that*?

As we'll see, many believe it to be essential. But the evidence is more mixed. I am going to concede that there are facets of intimate life where empathy does add something of value. But on balance, my conclusion here will be consistent with the overall theme of this book: It often does more harm than good.

Empathy has many champions, but one of the most thoughtful is Simon Baron-Cohen. We've already encountered his concerns about decision makers who lack empathy. But he also argues for the benefits of high empathy in personal relationships.

Plausibly enough, he assumes that people differ in how empathic they are, and he posits an empathy bell curve. It starts at Level 0, where a person feels no empathy at all, as with some psychopaths and narcissists. And it runs all the way to Level 6, the point at which an individual is "continuously focused on other people's feelings . . . in a constant state of hyperarousal, so that other people are never off their radar."

We don't have a name for such Level 6 people, and there's not as much research into them as for Level 0 people, so, absent the research, Baron-Cohen provides a sketch of one such Level 6 individual:

> Hannah is a psychotherapist who has a natural gift for tuning into how others are feeling. As soon as you walk into her living room, she is already reading your face, your gait, your posture. The first thing she asks you is "How are you?" but this is no perfunctory platitude. Her intonation—even before you have taken off your coat—suggests an invitation to confide, to disclose, to share. Even if you just answer with a short phrase, your tone of voice reveals to her your inner emotional state, and she quickly follows up your answer with "You sound a bit sad. What's happened to upset you?"

Before you know it, you are opening up to this wonderful listener, who interjects only to offer sounds of comfort and concern, to mirror how you feel, occasionally offering soothing words to boost you and make you feel valued. Hannah is not doing this because it is her job to do so. She is like this with her clients, her friends, and even people she has only just met. Hannah's friends feel cared for by her, and her friendships are built around sharing confidences and offering mutual support. She has an unstoppable drive to empathize.

It is easy to see what Baron-Cohen finds so impressive here. There is something moving about this portrayal. There are times when I would very much wish to have a Hannah in my life.

But thinking about Hannah leads us to raise some concerns with empathy. And to be fair, Baron-Cohen raises them too; in a footnote he mentions that there are studies on the risks of high empathy—but then he says that he doesn't think these risks would apply to someone like Hannah.

Well, let's see. Consider first what it must be like to be Hannah. Baron-Cohen is clear that her concern for other people isn't because she likes them or respects them. And it's not because she endorses some guiding principle of compassion and kindness. Rather, Hannah is compelled by her hyperarousal—her drive is *unstoppable*. Just as a selfish person might go through life concerned with his own pleasure and pain and indifferent to the pleasure and pain of others—99 for him and 1 for everyone else—Hannah is set up so that the experiences of others are always in her head—99 for everyone else and 1 for her.

This has a cost. It's no accident, in this regard, that Baron-Cohen chose a woman as his example. In a series of empirical and theoretical articles, Vicki Helgeson and Heidi Fritz explore sex differences in the propensity for what they call "unmitigated communion," defined as "an excessive concern with others and placing others' needs before one's own." To measure an individual's unmitigated communion, they developed a simple nine-item scale, where people rank themselves from "Strongly Disagree" to "Strongly Agree" on statements like

- "For me to be happy, I need others to be happy."
- "I can't say no when someone asks me for help."
- "I often worry about others' problems."

Women typically score higher than men on this scale—and Hannah would, I bet, score high indeed.

Being high in unmitigated communion is bad in many ways. In one study, people high on this scale were overprotective when a spouse had heart disease—as reported by both parties. They report asymmetrical relationships—they provide a lot of care to others but don't get much themselves. In fact, they are likely to say that they are uncomfortable being the recipients of support. Other studies show that if those high on the unmitigated communion scale hear about someone else's problem and are contacted a couple of days later, they are likely to report still being upset about it and suffering from intrusive thoughts.

Research with college students and with older adults finds that unmitigated communion is associated with being "overly nurturant, intrusive, and self-sacrificing." It is associated with the feeling that others don't like you and don't think well of you and with becoming upset when others don't want your help and don't take your advice. In laboratory studies, individuals with unmitigated communion are more bothered when a friend turns to someone else for help than when the friend doesn't get help at all.

High unmitigated communion is associated with poor adjustment, both physically and psychologically, and is linked to heart disease, diabetes, and cancer, perhaps because the focus on others keeps those high on the scale from attending to themselves.

Helgeson and Fritz speculate that the gender difference here explains women's greater propensity to anxiety and depression, a conclusion that meshes with the proposal by Barbara Oakley, who, drawing on work on "pathological altruism," notes, "It's surprising how many diseases and syndromes commonly seen in women seem to be related to women's generally stronger empathy for and focus on others."

The phrase "unmitigated communion" might make you wonder if the problem is with the "unmitigated" part, not the "communion" part. And indeed, the initial research into this area was motivated by the work of David Bakan, who discusses two central aspects of human nature: agency and communion. *Agency* emphasizes self and separation and is a stereotypically male trait. *Communion* emphasizes connection with people and is stereotypically female. Both have value, and both are needed to be psychologically complete.

Zooming in on communion—good communion, not the unmitigated type—there is a scale for this as well. (We psychologists do love our scales.) This involves rating yourself from 1 to 5 on traits such as:

- Helpful
- Aware of other's feelings
- Kind
- Understanding of others

Not surprisingly, scoring high on this scale is associated with all sorts of positive things, including good health.

So what's the difference between people who are high in communion (positive) and those who are high in unmitigated communion (negative)? Both sorts of people care about others. But communion corresponds to what we can call concern and compassion, while unmitigated communion ends up relating more to empathy or, more precisely, *empathic distress*—suffering at the suffering of others.

I don't think being high in unmitigated communion is exactly the same as being high in empathy. But they give rise to the same underlying vulnerability when it comes to interacting with other people. They lead to an overly personal distress that interferes with one's life.

The concern about Baron-Cohen's hypothetical Hannah is not that she cares about other people. You should care about other people. Putting aside the obvious point that some degree of caring for others is morally right, it turns out that altruistic action is associated with all sorts of good physical and psychological outcomes, including a boost in both short-term mood and long-term happiness—if you want to get happy, helping other people is an excellent way to do so.

Rather, Hannah's problem is that her caring is driven by her receptivity to suffering. She appears to be high in unmitigated communion. The research that I just reviewed suggests that this is harmful in the long run.

This concern takes us in a new direction. My argument in previous chapters has been that empathy, because of its spotlight nature, is a poor moral guide. It is biased, it is innumerate, and so on. But here I am suggesting that empathy can also have negative consequences for those who experience it.

You probably have never heard about unmitigated communion before, but the idea that you can feel too much of the suffering of others will be familiar. This is sometimes called "burnout," a word that was coined in the 1970s. But it's not a new insight; the idea has many origins, including, to my surprise, in Buddhist theology.

I first learned this from a discussion I had with Matthieu Ricard, the Buddhist monk and neuroscientist described by many as "the happiest man on Earth." Our meeting was by chance—we were checking into a hotel on the outskirts of London for a conference where we were both speaking. I recognized him at the front desk (saffron robes, beatific smile, hard to miss) and introduced myself, and we got together later for tea.

It was an interesting meeting. He really does exude inner peace, and he told me that he spends months of each year in total solitude, getting deep pleasure from this. (It was this conversation that has led me to adopt meditative practices myself, however unevenly.) At one point he politely asked me what I was working on. Now it seemed at the time that telling someone like Ricard that you're writing a book against empathy was like telling an orthodox rabbi that you're writing a book in favor of shellfish, and I felt awkward describing this project. But I did, and his reaction to my empathy trash talk surprised me.

He didn't find it shocking; rather, he found it obviously correct and went on to describe how well it meshes with both Buddhist philosophy and his own collaborative research with Tania Singer, a prominent neuroscientist.

Consider first the life of a bodhisattva, an enlightened person who vows not to pass into Nirvana, choosing instead to stay in the normal cycle of life and death to help the unenlightened masses. How is a bodhisattva to live?

In his book on Buddhist moral philosophy, Charles Goodman notes that Buddhist texts distinguish between "sentimental compassion," which corresponds to what we would call empathy, and "great compassion," which is what we would simply call "compassion." The first is to be avoided, as it "exhausts the bodhisattva." It's the second that is worth pursuing. Great compassion is more distanced and reserved, and can be sustained indefinitely.

This distinction between empathy and compassion is critical for the argument I've been making throughout this book. And it is supported by neuroscience research. In a review article, Tania Singer and Olga Klimecki describe how they make sense of this distinction: "In contrast to empathy, compassion does not mean sharing the suffering of the other: rather, it is characterized by feelings of warmth, concern and care for the other, as well as a strong motivation to improve the other's well-being. Compassion is feeling for and not feeling with the other."

The neurological difference between the two was explored in a series of fMRI studies that used Ricard as a subject. While in the scanner, Ricard was asked to engage in various types of compassion meditation directed toward people who are suffering. To the surprise of the investigators, his meditative states did not activate those parts of the brain associated with empathic distress—those that are normally activated by nonmeditators when they think about others' pain. And Ricard's experience was pleasant and invigorating. Once out of the magnet, Ricard described it as: "a warm positive state associated with a strong prosocial motivation."

He was then asked to put himself in an empathic state and was scanned while doing so. Now the appropriate empathy circuits were activated: His brain looked the same as those of nonmeditators who were asked to think about the pain of others. Ricard later described the experience: "The empathic sharing . . . very quickly became intolerable to me and I felt emotionally exhausted, very similar to being burned out. After nearly an hour of empathic resonance, I was given the choice to engage in compassion or to finish scanning. Without the slightest hesitation, I agreed to continue scanning with compassion meditation, because I felt so drained after the empathic resonance."

One sees a similar contrast in ongoing experiments led by Singer in which normal people—nonmeditators—were trained to experience either empathy or compassion. In empathy training, people were instructed to try to feel what others were feeling. In compassion training—sometimes called "loving-kindness meditation"—the goal is to feel positive and warm thoughts toward a series of imagined persons, starting with someone close to you and moving to strangers and, perhaps, to enemies.

There is a neural difference: Empathy training led to increased activation in the insula and anterior cingulate cortex (both of which we discussed in relation to the neuroscience-of-empathy studies in an earlier chapter). Compassion training led to activation in other parts of the brain, such as the medial orbitofrontal cortex and ventral striatum.

There is also a practical difference. When people were asked to empathize with those who were suffering, they found it unpleasant. Compassion training, in contrast, led to better feelings on the part of the meditator and kinder behavior toward others.

The contrast here between empathy and compassion should look familiar. When I described what's wrong with unmitigated communion, I drew upon findings suggesting that the culprit was distress: Unmitigated communion makes you suffer when faced with those who are suffering, which imposes costs on yourself and makes you less effective at helping. This might also explain what's so bad about empathy training and why compassion training is superior. In a summary of her research, Singer makes the same point in rather more careful language and then explores broader implications:

> When experienced chronically, empathic distress most likely gives rise to negative health outcomes. On the other hand, compassionate responses are based on positive, other-oriented feelings and the activation of prosocial motivation and behavior. Given the potentially detrimental effects of empathic distress, the finding of existing plasticity of adaptive social emotions is encouraging, especially as compassion training not only promotes prosocial behavior, but also augments positive affect and resilience, which in turn fosters better coping with stressful situations. This opens up many opportunities for the targeted development of adaptive social emotions and motivation, which can be particularly beneficial for persons working in helping professions or in stressful environments in general.

This connects nicely with the conclusions of David DeSteno and his colleagues, who find, in controlled experimental studies, that being trained in mindfulness meditation (as opposed to a control condition where people are trained in other cognitive skills) makes people kinder to others and more willing to help. DeSteno and his colleagues argue that mindfulness meditation "reduces activation of the brain networks associated with simulating the feelings of people in distress, in favor of networks associated with feelings of social affiliation." He approvingly quotes the Buddhist scholar Thupten Jinpa: "meditation-based training enables practitioners to move quickly from feeling the distress of others to acting with compassion to alleviate it."

Less empathy, more kindness.

These studies bear on the claims of those psychologists and neuroscientists who believe that compassion and empathy are necessarily intertwined. In critical responses to an earlier article I wrote, Leonardo Christov-Moore and Marco Iacoboni claimed that "affective empathy is a precursor to compassion," and Lynn E. O'Connor and Jack W. Berry wrote, "We can't feel compassion without first feeling emotional empathy. Indeed compassion is the extension of emotional empathy by means of cognitive processes."

As I've mentioned a few times by now, it's hard to know what to make of these claims, given all of the everyday instances in which we care for people and help them without engaging in emotional empathy. I can worry about a child who is afraid of a thunderstorm and pick her up and comfort her without experiencing her fear in the slightest. I can be concerned about starving people and try to support them without having any vicarious experience of starving. And now the research we just discussed supports an even stronger conclusion. Not only can compassion and kindness exist independently of empathy, they are sometimes opposed. Sometimes we are better people if we suppress our empathic feelings.

These worries about the negative effects of empathy might be surprising to those involved in the training of doctors. There is a lot of concern about studies that find a decline in empathy in medical students. Empathy has been named an "essential learning objective" by the American Association of Medical Colleges, and there is a special focus on empathy training in medical schools.

For the most part, I'm all for this. As we've seen, people often use the term *empathy* to include all sorts of good things, and most of what goes on in the name of empathy training in medical school is hard to object to, such as encouraging doctors to listen to patients, to take time with them, and to show respect. It's only when we think about empathy in a more literal sense that we run into problems.

Christine Montross, a surgeon, weighs in on the risks of empathy: "If, while listening to the grieving mother's raw and unbearable description of her son's body in the morgue, I were to imagine my own son in his place, I would be incapacitated. My ability to attend to my patient's psychiatric needs would be derailed by my own devastating sorrow. Similarly, if I were brought in by ambulance to the trauma bay of my local emergency department and required immediate surgery to save my life, I would not want the trauma surgeon on call to pause to empathize with my pain and suffering."

Montross's remarks were sparked by an article I wrote where I talked about problems with empathy in medical contexts.

Soon after this article was published, I received the following letter from another doctor, this time an emergency physician, which I am quoting with her permission:

> I have always felt that I am very empathetic, and that that has been both a blessing and a curse in my work. I have struggled with burn-out for years. . . . I have felt that I was being less than helpful to my patients if I shut down my empathetic response to their pain. This really got me into trouble when I was part of a disaster medical relief team sent to the World Trade Center site. We were there at the beginning of November, so there were no living victims of the attacks to care for, only the crews that were digging up bodies. . . . I not only opened myself up to trying to be there and feel the pain with the workers there, but I also tried to really take in my surroundings and feel the horror and the loss around me. I felt it was somehow immoral not to. One day I was way too successful at being empathetic in that way, and it was more than I could take. My mind just couldn't handle it. It was like trying to drink from a firehose, and I was drowning.

She added that the research I described concerning the distinction between empathy and compassion—some of the same research described above—helped her appreciate that the problems she had with empathy do not make her a bad person:

> It is a relief to know that I am not somehow shirking my humanity to not feel the pain of families who are making end of life decisions for a loved one, or who are getting the news of a loved one's death, or people who I am telling that they

have cancer or a fetus with a malformed head. It is a nice idea that I can actively work to shut down my emotional response without losing my compassion.

These problems with empathy are familiar enough to those in the profession. A friend of mine who is a pediatric surgeon told me of two medical students who had to shift to other specialties because of the stress of working with parents and children in severe circumstances. One study found that nursing students who were especially prone to empathy spent less time providing care to patients and more time seeking out help from other hospital personnel, presumably because of how aversive they found it to deal with people who were suffering.

The risks of empathy are perhaps most obvious with therapists, who have to continually deal with people who are depressed, anxious, deluded, and often in severe emotional pain. There is a rich theoretical discussion among therapists, particularly those of a psychoanalytic orientation, about the complex interpersonal relationships between therapists and their clients. But anyone who thinks that it's important for a therapist to feel depressed or anxious while dealing with depressed or anxious people is missing the point of therapy.

Actually, therapy would be an impossible job for many of us because of our inability to shut down our empathic responses. But good therapists are unusual in this regard. A friend of mine is a clinical psychologist with a busy schedule, working for several hours at a stretch, with one client leaving and the next coming in. This would kill me. I find it exhausting to spend even a short time with someone who is depressed or anxious. But my friend finds it exhilarating. She is engaged by her clients' problems, interested in the challenges that arise, and excited by the possibility of improving their lives.

Her description reminded me of a discussion by the writer and surgeon Atul Gawande about the attitudes of "tenderness and aestheticism" that good surgeons feel toward their patients, treating them with respect but seeing them also as problems that need to be solved. Freud himself made a similar analogy: "I cannot advise my colleagues too urgently to model themselves during psycho-analytic treatment on the surgeon, who puts aside all his feelings, even his human sympathy, and concentrates his mental forces on the single aim of performing the operations as skillfully as possible."

My friend does get into her clients' heads, of course—she would be useless if she couldn't—but she doesn't feel what they feel. She employs understanding and caring, not empathy.

I've looked so far at the effects of empathy on the empathizer. But what about those who are empathized with? People in distress plainly want respect, compassion, kindness, and attention—but do they want empathy? Do they benefit from it?

A few years ago, my uncle, a man I respected and loved very much, was undergoing treatment for cancer. While he went to hospitals and rehabilitation centers, I watched him interact with many doctors and talked to him about what he thought of them. He appreciated when doctors listened to him and worked to understand his situation; he resonated to this sort of "cognitive empathy." He appreciated as well those doctors who expressed compassion and caring and warmth.

But what about the more emotional side of empathy? Here

it's more complicated. He seemed to get the most from doctors who *didn't* feel as he did, who were calm when he was anxious, confident when he was uncertain. And he was particularly appreciative of certain virtues that have little directly to do with empathy, such as competence, honesty, professionalism, and certainly respect.

A similar point is made by Leslie Jamison in the opening essay of her collection, *The Empathy Exams.* Jamison describes a period in which she worked as a simulated patient for medical students, rating them on their skills, with one item being Checklist item 31: "Voiced empathy for my situation/problem." But when she draws on her own personal experiences with doctors, she finds herself more skeptical about empathy's centrality.

She tells about how she met with a doctor who was cold and unsympathetic to her concerns, and talks about the pain that it caused her. But she also describes, with gratitude, another doctor who kept a reassuring distance and objectivity: "I didn't need him to be my mother—even for a day—I only needed him to know what he was doing. . . . His calmness didn't make me feel abandoned, it made me feel secure. . . . I wanted to look at him and see the opposite of my fear, not its echo."

Now I've cited both Christine Montross and Leslie Jamison in support of my arguments for the limits of empathy, but to be fair, both of them also defend empathy to some degree. After the passage I cited above, where Montross talks about why she wouldn't want to feel too much empathy for a patient and why she wouldn't want a too-empathic doctor, she steps back a bit: "Still, in most of the interactions physicians have with patients in everyday medicine—indeed in my own clinical work—it is easy to see how a reasonable amount of empathy can be beneficial, for both parties. Patients feel heard and understood. Doctors appreciate their patients' concerns and feel compelled to do as much as possible to alleviate their suffering."

And after describing the value of the doctor who kept more of a distance, Jamison goes on to add: "I appreciated the care of a doctor who didn't simply echo my fears. But without empathy, this doctor wouldn't have been able to offer the care I ended up appreciating. He needed to inhabit my feelings long enough to offer an alternative to them and to help dissolve them by offering information, guidance, and reassurance."

I agree with a lot of this. It makes sense that concern and understanding are important. But I think it's possible to have concern and understanding while maintaining an emotional distance, without the doctor or therapist having to "inhabit" the patient's feelings. I think it's actually better when this distance is present, both for the patient and for the doctor.

One might reasonably object that caring just doesn't work this way. Perhaps the only way one can truly understand what someone is going through is to feel what they are feeling. The sort of intellectual understanding that I've been talking about so far just isn't enough.

When people make this argument, though, I think they are getting distracted by a different issue. They are compelled by the idea that you can't truly understand something without having experienced it yourself. A good therapist, one might argue, should understand what it's like to be depressed and anxious and lonely—and this means that he or she must have at one point felt depressed and anxious and lonely. These are the sorts of experiences—what Laurie Paul calls "transformative experiences"—that you have to undergo yourself in order to know what they're like. Imagination isn't enough. There's just no substitute for the real thing.

Frank Jackson makes this point through a famous thought experiment (one expanded upon in the wonderful science fiction/horror movie, *Ex Machina*). Jackson tells the story of Mary, a brilliant scientist, who has spent her life stuck in a black-and-white room, with a black-and-white television monitor. Mary studies human perception and comes to know everything about the neuroscience of seeing color. She knows the wavelengths of the colors, she knows what neurons fire when people see green, she knows that people describe both blood and stop signs as "red," she knows what happens when you mix paints—she knows all the facts about colors. But aside from the black and white of the room and what she can see of her own body, she has no experience of color.

Now imagine that Mary leaves the room for the first time and looks up to see a bright blue sky. Most people's intuition here is that she now knows something that she didn't before. In the language of philosophy, there is some novel qualitative experience—*qualia*—that exists above and beyond nonperceptual knowledge. Jackson takes this as having some strong metaphysical implications about the nature of the mind, and there is much debate about this, but a more modest interpretation is that his thought experiment shows that you can learn some things through experience that cannot be appreciated in any other way. You have to be there. To know what it's like to see blue, Mary has to see blue.

To bring it back to our current concerns, certain real experiences might be indispensable for a therapist. From the standpoint of the patient, it can be comforting to talk to someone who knows just how you are feeling. From the standpoint of the therapist, figuring out how to help the patient surely benefits from appreciating what the patient is going through.

But this is not an argument in favor of empathy. To get this appreciation, you don't need to actually mirror another's feelings. There is a world of difference, after all, between understanding the misery of the person who is talking to you because you have felt misery in the past, even though now you are calm, and understanding the misery of the person who is talking to you because you are mirroring them and feeling their misery *right now*. The first, which doesn't involve empathy in any sense, just understanding, has all the advantages of the second and none of its costs.

What about our relationships with those we love? We've been discussing doctors and therapists—individuals who have relationships with people that are in certain respects intimate. But still, there is supposed to be some distance there. These professionals typically work with multiple individuals and do so at least in part because they are paid. And then they go home at the end of the day.

Friends and family are different. They *are* home with you; they don't have the same boundaries. What works for strangers might not work for these more intimate relationships.

There's a similar concern about the "great compassion" explored in certain schools of Buddhism. One might worry that it is incompatible with the partiality that is an essential part of close relationships. This is summed up in an old joke:

—Did you hear about the Buddhist vacuum cleaner?
—It comes with no attachments.

As we consider what we want in close relationships, let's get the obvious out of the way. Most people, I assume, want to be loved and understood and cared about. Indeed, we want our friends and family to care about us *more* than they care about other people. For many, this is just what it means to be in a close and intimate relationship.

Such caring means that our feelings will often be in synchrony with those we love. It would certainly be unnerving if someone I love were happy when I was miserable and miserable when I was happy. This would cause me to question how much this person loved me back.

But that isn't because I want empathic mirroring. If someone cares about me, my sadness should make her sad, my happiness should make her happy. If my niece is delighted because she just won a scholarship, this will make me happy, but not because I'm vicariously experiencing her pleasure. Instead it's because I love her and want her to do well. Indeed, I might be just as happy if I heard about her good fortune before she did, so that no mirroring could conceivably take place.

There are also times when feelings should diverge. This is in part because people in a normal relationship have some autonomy and independence and in part because if you care for another, you shouldn't always want to mirror that person's moods. As Cicero said about the merits of friendship—but he could just as well have been talking about close relationships in general—it "improves happiness and abates misery, by the doubling of our joy and the dividing of our grief." I would prefer that those who care about me greet my panic with calm and my gloom with good cheer.

The intricacies here are nicely explored by Adam Smith. I

won't pretend that Smith is my ally in my antiempathy crusade, as he often argues for empathy's centrality in human affairs. But regardless, he is a savvy interpreter of social interaction and has a particularly subtle analysis of the role of empathy in friendship.

Smith begins by talking about a virtue of empathy. If you're anxious, it pays to be empathic with a calm friend because this will make you calm and help you make sense of your situation: "The mind, therefore, is rarely so disturbed, but that the company of a friend will restore it to some degree of tranquility and sedateness. The breast is, in some measure, calmed and composed the moment we come into his presence. We are immediately put in mind of the light in which he will view our situation, and we begin to view it ourselves in the same light; for the effect of sympathy is instantaneous."

Smith inverts the sort of empathic distress scenario that we've worried about in the therapeutic context, where a calm person (the therapist) meets an upset person (the client), and through empathy the calm person becomes upset. Here, the calm person meets the upset person and the upset person becomes calm. This is a better model for what should go on in therapy—the trick, then, is not for the therapist to have empathy; it's for the patient to have it.

It gets more complicated when we encounter a very happy friend. We're capable of empathizing with "small joys," says Smith, but someone who has been transported to great fortune, "may be assured that the congratulations of his best friends are not all of them perfectly sincere." Envy can block empathy. If you won the prize that I have always coveted, it's hard for me to fully share your joy; my envy and my empathy fight it out.

Your happy friend can best make you happy when envy

doesn't apply. This can occur when the boundaries of the self somehow expand to include the happy person, so that his accomplishment feels like my accomplishment. This most easily happens with the accomplishments of one's children, perhaps, but it can also apply when we see people as bringing credit to our communities. When Daniel Kahneman won a Nobel Prize, I was delighted because he is a fellow psychologist; when Robert Schiller won one, I was delighted because he is from Yale and, more important, lives on my street, eight houses down from my own. So, in some possibly pathetic way, their great accomplishments became my own.

Envy can also be reduced if the accomplishment is in a domain that we don't care about—I won't envy you getting top prize for your heirloom tomatoes, because I don't like to garden. (Though even here I might envy how impressed people are with you.)

Because of the risk of envy, Smith's advice to someone who has sudden great fortune is to try to keep the joy to himself, not make a big thing out of it, keep humble, and be extra kind to his friends. Good advice, I think.

I'll add, by the way, that Smith's discussion of those cases when we do respond well to the "small joys" runs the risk of blurring two things. Our positive response might be due to genuine empathy (what Smith would call "sympathy"). But alternatively, the positive response might just be because I care for you, so assuming that I can override envy, your good fortune makes me happy as well.

This second nonempathic response is probably more common. Imagine that I learn that my good friend has fallen in love, and this fills my heart with joy. But it's not because I'm feeling the giddiness and excitement of a new romance. No, I'm feeling good simply because I like my friend. Even in this mundane example, we have to be careful not to overstate the role of empathy.

Consider finally our dealings with a friend who is sad. We are capable of exercising empathy here, but there are reasons why we might choose not to.

One is that you might think he or she is sad for a silly reason. As mentioned earlier, Smith gives the example of someone who tells you how annoyed he is that "his brother hummed a tune all the time he himself was telling a story." So he's upset, but you're not, because you find this ridiculous. You might actually find this pretty entertaining—a reaction that Smith calls "a malice in mankind."

More generally, we just don't like empathizing with the sad. It makes us sad, and we have enough problems of our own! Smith puts this more eloquently: "Nature, it seems, when she loaded us with our own sorrows, thought that they were enough, and therefore did not command us to take any further share in those of others, than what was necessary to prompt us to relieve them." Smith suggests that sad people should be aware of how unwilling people are to empathize with them and should be reticent in sharing their sadness with others.

Now I admit that there is something odd about getting life advice from Adam Smith (though there is an excellent book called *How Adam Smith Can Change Your Life*). Although he had close relationships with friends and was a wonderful son to his mother, there is no evidence that he ever had any close romantic or sexual relationship with man or woman. (I was once at the dinner after a morality conference, surrounded by Smith experts, and their heated argument was over whether he died a virgin.) But still, his caution about oversharing and his demands for reticence fit well with the arguments in this chapter and also sit well with my own cold and repressed Canadian heart.

Smith had no children. While friends, lovers, and spouses are among the closest relationships, the tie between parents and children is special. From the perspective of evolution, there is nothing that matters more. Our children are the primary means through which we pass on our genes, so our sentiments have evolved to nurture this relationship. Indeed, many scholars have argued that empathy itself has evolved for the purpose of parenting—in particular, to guide the mother and child to establish a synchrony so that they come to feel one another's experiences, allowing the mother to better take care of the child.

What role, then, does empathy play in good parenting? An obvious starting point here is that good parents understand and love their children. (This has to be the most banal sentence of this book.) Nobody wants to parent like Betty Draper, a character in the period drama *Mad Men*.

> **Child:** "I'm bored."
> **Betty:** "Go bang your head against the wall."
> **Child:** "Mom?"
> **Betty:** "Only boring people get bored."

But good parenting also requires an appreciation that the long-term goals of a child do not always correspond to his or her short-term wants. My worst moments as a father aren't when I don't care; they're when I care too much, when I cannot disengage from my children's frustration or pain.

It would be fair to object that understanding and compassion, even love, are not all children want. Sometimes they may want the more intimate connection that empathy can provide. My colleague Stephen Darwall put this nicely in a discussion of what it is like when we are "accountable" to another person: "we put ourselves in their hands, give them a special standing to hold us answerable, and make ourselves vulnerable, through projective empathy, to their feelings and attitudes, not just as the latter's targets, but as feelings we can bring home to ourselves and share."

Elaborating on this point, Darwall discusses an example from Michael Slote. Imagine a father whose daughter enjoys stamp collecting. It might be nice for the father to tell her that he approves of the hobby and that he respects it. But wouldn't it be better if he could share her excitement? "The father who becomes 'infected' with his daughter's interest in and enthusiasm about stamp collecting is showing a kind of (unself-conscious) respect for his daughter."

Moving back to adults now, there are numerous cases where you want someone to feel as you do, where you want them to feel empathic toward *you*. Adam Smith's calm friend might want his agitated buddy to catch some of his calmness. Other examples range from the religious (If only you could know, as I do, what it's like to be loved by God), to the sexual (I wish you could feel how good that feels), to the mundane (Dude, you just have to try these tacos—they're awesome!).

It's not all positive feelings, though. Often we want others to feel our pain. After all, we know that feeling empathy for an individual makes you more likely to help them—the studies that I reviewed in a previous chapter are decisive here. So if I'm suffering and I want your help, I can try to evoke your empathy. There is some risk here, though. You have to hit a sweet spot because, as we've seen, too much empathy can be paralyzing. Someone who might otherwise have helped me might feel my pain, find it too much to bear, and walk away.

There is another, very different reason to want others to feel your pain. When people who are wronged describe their feelings toward those who harmed them, they often say that they want them to suffer, but sometimes they say something more precise— they want the wrongdoer to feel the same pain as the victim.

Consider apologies. When people list what makes a good apology, they often include empathic resonance on the part of the wrongdoer. One list of criteria for good apologies, by Heidi Howkins Lockwood, includes this:

> **It should be a sincere and non-obsequious display of empathy and/or affect:**
> Some victims point to an affective element that must be present for an apology to be "real" or effective. . . . Perhaps even more important than the affect is empathy. As one survivor of an instance of sexual misconduct in philosophy said to me last fall, "I don't want him [the offender] to suffer; there's already been enough of that. I just wish I could somehow make him see what I've been through." To *see* or *feel* what a victim has been through requires an empathetic and vivid reimagining of both the offense and the context of offense from the point of view of the offended.

In *On Apology*, Aaron Lazare offers a similar sentiment: "what makes an apology work is the exchange of shame and power between the offender and the offended. By apologizing, you take the shame of your offense and redirect it to yourself."

Why "a vivid reimagining"? Why an "exchange" of shame? Lockwood says that the victim she spoke with doesn't want the perpetrator to suffer, but I think a more honest reckoning is that she doesn't *merely* want him to suffer. It's unsatisfying having someone who has victimized you feel no pain at all, but it's also not enough for that person to feel pain of a sort that's unrelated to the victimization—ideally, the sexual harasser should feel what it's like to be the victim of sexual harassment. If he suffers because his child falls ill or his house burns down, it might be satisfying, but it's not quite the same.

Why is this symmetry so important? One consideration relates to something we've discussed before, which is the connection between understanding and experience. The victim might believe both that a sincere apology requires the perpetrator understanding what he or she did wrong . . . and that truly understanding what one did wrong requires having the experience yourself.

Then there is the wish to restore balance. Pamela Hieronymi puts it like this: "A past wrong against you, standing in your history without apology, atonement, retribution, punishment, restitution, condemnation, or anything else that might recognize it as a wrong, makes a claim. It says, in effect, that you can be treated in this way, and that such treatment is acceptable." Those practices she lists, starting with apologies, serve to repair the victim's status—to use that lovely legal expression, they serve to make the victim whole again.

From this perspective, an apology involves an acknowledgment that it is unacceptable to harm someone without just cause. For this to work, it has to be somehow costly; you need to know that the person means it, so some suffering is needed. Empathy allows for a perfect eye-for-an-eye correspondence, where the perpetrator experiences the very same suffering as the victim.

We've talked here about the role that empathy plays in certain personal aspects of our lives, looking at the sorts of relationships that therapists and doctors have with their patients, at friendship, and at parenting. We've treated this as a separate issue from the question that occupied the first part of the book, which focused on dealing with strangers, as in public policy and decisions over charitable giving.

It would certainly be simpler if we could keep these issues separate—if there were two moralities, one for home and one for the outside world. But any sharp distinction quickly collapses because there is only so much to go around. If I have a hundred dollars and decide to give it to one of my sons so he can buy books for school, that's a hundred dollars that's not going to help children who are going blind in Africa. If I get to decide who to hire as a research assistant in my lab and my friend asks me to hire his daughter, my loyalty to my friend will clash with any fair and neutral process for choosing the candidates.

Not everyone sees this tension. One intellectual wrote with great admiration about Noam Chomsky, about his work for various social causes, his intellectual courage, his tireless advocacy for the weak, how he has devoted his life to helping others, and so on, but then added this remark: "he is an absolutely faithful person, he will never betray you. He's constitutionally incapable of betrayal. To the point that he will defend friends even though I think he knows they're wrong, but he won't ever betray you."

But you can't have both. Chomsky can't both be intellectually robust and at the same time defend friends at all costs. Our parochial affection for those around us—the affection that is driven by empathic feelings—is often at war with the sort of impartiality that is at the core of all moral systems.

Some resolve this tension by saying, essentially, to hell with impartial morality. In a recent book, Stephen Asma argues for the moral importance of kinship and loyalty, the importance of favoring those who are close to you. He is quite aware that this clashes with justice and fairness: His book is called *Against Fairness*. (Not to pick on Asma here, but can you *imagine* a more obnoxious title?)

Asma begins by describing a time when he was on a panel on ethics, along with a priest and a communist. At some point he said, to the shock of his fellow participants, "I would strangle everyone in this room if it somehow prolonged my son's life." He was kidding as he said it, but during the drive home, he realized that he believed it. He would save his son's life at the cost of others, and he wasn't ashamed of it. He writes, "The utilitarian demand—that I should always maximize the greatest good for the greatest number—seemed reasonable to me in my twenties but made me laugh after my son was born."

Asma is in good company here. Blood is thicker than water—and many see something ridiculous, or worse, about anyone who doesn't know this. In his discussion of Gandhi's autobiography, George Orwell expresses admiration for Gandhi's courage but is repelled by Gandhi's rejection of special relationships—of friends and family, of sexual and romantic love. Orwell describes this as "inhuman," and goes on to say: "The essence of being human is that one does not seek perfection, that one is sometimes willing to commit sins for the sake of loyalty, that one does not push asceticism to the point where it makes friendly intercourse impossible, and that one is prepared in the end to be defeated and broken up by life, which is the inevitable price of fastening one's love upon other human individuals."

To go back to the Dickensian discussion from earlier in this chapter, Charles Dickens had an immense social conscience — but he would ridicule those who lacked special feelings for those close to them. His examples include Thomas Gradgrind, the extreme utilitarian, and Mrs. Jellyby, who we meet in a chapter of *Bleak House* titled "Telescopic Philanthropy" — she cares about those in faraway lands but she neglects her family: Her son has his head stuck through the railings, while she prattles on about the natives of Borrioboola-Gha.

Others, though, would say to hell with special relationships. It is wrong, many people believe, to treat people differently because of the color of their skin or because of their sex or their sexual orientation. Some, like Peter Singer, take this further and argue that it is wrong to favor members of our own species and wrong as well to favor people just because they are physically close to us. Along the lines of the arguments I've been making here, Singer argues that relying on our gut feelings can make us less moral and more partial.

As an intelligent utilitarian, Singer appreciates that some parochial actions and attitudes might serve to maximize overall happiness. If you and I both have babies, they are most likely to survive if I take care of mine and you take care of yours. But a utilitarian like Singer — in direct opposition to someone like

Asma—would insist that this bias has no intrinsic value. Like our appetite for punishment, our relatively greater concern for those close to us might be a necessary evil.

Singer is in good company when he dismisses the intrinsic value of intimate relationships, and it's not just Gandhi. As Larissa MacFarquhar points out, Abraham was ready to sacrifice his beloved son; Buddha abandoned his family; Jesus was adamant that in order to become his disciple, one must "hate his own father and mother and wife and children and brothers and sisters, yes, and even his own life."

So there are two broader perspectives here, one which sees the parochial force of sentiments like empathy as something to be applauded, something that makes us human, and another that sees it as a moral wrong turn.

I said at the start of this book that my argument against empathy wouldn't be that it violates my notion of right and wrong, it's that it violates yours. It has effects that almost everyone will agree are wrong. If I were to endorse a hard-core impartiality position, I would be breaking my word. Many people would say that we have every right to care about those close to us over those far away, and if empathy guides us in this direction, more power to it. Most people, I imagine, would choose Orwell and Asma over Gandhi and Singer.

I am, to some extent, one of these people. I resonate to Dickens's mockery. I could never take seriously people who refuse to take long flights to see those they love because of worries about contributing to climate change. Or even those who put their children into a public school that they know to be terrible even though they can easily afford a private school, just out of a broader principle of common good. Even when it comes to charity, I am not a good utilitarian. I give far too little to charity, and some of the charities that I do give to, such as Special Olympics, were chosen by accidents of sentiment, not through a thoughtful and impartial calculation. I eat meat. I retain both my kidneys, though I understand that I only need one and there are others who could really use my spare. And so on. Like Asma, and like most everyone I know, I care much more for me and mine than I care for strangers.

But my partiality has limits, and I bet yours does too. If I were hurrying home to join my family for dinner and I passed a lost child, I would help the child find his parents, even if it made me a bit late and caused some mild distress to those I love. So strangers have *some* weight.

One of the hardest moral projects that any person faces concerns the proper balance here. How much money and time—and attention and emotional energy—should we spend on ourselves, on those close to us, and on strangers? MacFarquhar notes that there is something taboo about this question. That someone who "even asks himself how much he should do for his family and how much for strangers—weighing the two together on the same balance—may seem already a step too far." But the situations in everyday life force us to confront the problem, to balance self versus family versus stranger. If you're mathematically inclined, you can think of it in terms of the following formula:

$$\text{Self} + \text{Close People} + \text{Strangers} = 100\%$$

Now fill in the numbers. Someone who had Self = 100% would be a pure egoist, and would surely be a monster; someone who had Self = 0% would be some sort of crazy saint. Throughout history, many people have had Strangers = 0%; in my last book, *Just Babies*, I argued that this is the default mode of human nature. But I can't imagine that many people have it *now*; few people would let a stranger die—at least someone in front of them—if a rescue cost them very little. So I know what the numbers *shouldn't* be. But I don't know what they are, or how one could find out, or even whether this is the best way to frame the problem.

I've conceded the importance of some amount of partiality here, the value of giving family and friends some special weight. So it might look as if I've opened up the door, perhaps just a bit, for empathy.

But not really. Yes, empathy is biased and parochial—but in a stupid way. Even if we decide that certain individuals are worthy of special treatment, even here empathy lets us down, because empathy is driven by immediate considerations, making us too-permissive parents and too-clingy friends. It's not just that it fails us as a tool for fair and impartial moral judgment, then, it's often a failure with intimate relationships. We can often do much better.

Empathy as the Foundation of Morality

Perhaps empathy is like milk. Adults don't need milk; we do fine without it. But babies need milk to grow.

Many of my fellow psychologists—and many philosophers, and many parents—see empathy as the developmental core of morality. They see babies as highly empathic creatures— empathic in the Adam Smith sense of naturally resonating to the feelings of others. As babies grow, this empathy-based morality gradually expands and gets more abstract, so that ultimately there is caring without stepping into others' shoes, as well as the capacity for objective moral reasoning.

One appeal of this view is its simplicity. To explain morality, all you need to attribute to babies is a single thing—the spark of empathy, the capacity to feel the feelings of others. Everything else follows from this spark. This is a pleasingly minimalist solution and it will appeal to those who are loath to attribute too much mental richness to such a tiny brain.

This empathy-first account was endorsed, in somewhat different forms, by two of the great philosophers of the Scottish Enlightenment: Adam Smith and David Hume. And it's been endorsed as well by many contemporary developmental psychologists. Martin Hoffman, for instance, defines empathy in a way that fits with how we are talking about it here—"an affective response more appropriate to another's situation than one's own"—and presents a detailed theory of its development, arguing that empathy is the foundation of morality. For him, empathy is "the spark of human concern for others, the glue that makes social life possible."

If this turns out to be right, it need not clash with the arguments I've been making so far. Even if empathy is foundational for children, it might be useless or even detrimental for adults. One could write a book called *Against Milk*, after all, while acknowledging that milk is just fine for babies.

I'm against empathy, but I do believe that people feel compassion. We want to help others and want to employ our hearts and minds to achieve good ends. There are those who doubt even this, who reject the notion that we possess any sort of kind or compassionate motivation. They think that people are ultimately selfish and self-interested.

Of course, these cynics have to concede that we sometimes help others, even strangers. We give to charity, donate blood, post helpful reviews on Internet sites, and so on. But the claim is that there is always an ulterior motive. We wish to improve our reputations, or get others to help us in the future, or attract mates and friends. Or perhaps we want to feel good about ourselves, or go to heaven after we die. Our intentions are never pure, and we're fooling ourselves if we think they are. As Michael Ghiselin put it: "Scratch an altruist, and watch a hypocrite bleed."

Many brilliant people have come to this conclusion. The story goes that Thomas Hobbes was walking through London with a friend when Hobbes stopped to give money to a beggar. The friend was surprised and pointed out to Hobbes that he had long argued for the fundamentally egoistic nature of humanity. Hobbes replied that there was no contradiction. He was motivated by pure self-interest—giving made him feel better; it was painful for him to see the beggar suffer.

Then there is this story of Abraham Lincoln, as it was reported in a newspaper at the time:

> Mr. Lincoln once remarked to a fellow-passenger on an old-time mud-coach that all men were prompted by selfishness in doing good. His fellow-passenger was antagonizing this position when they were passing over a corduroy bridge that spanned a slough. As they crossed this bridge they espied an old razor-backed sow on the bank making a terrible noise because her pigs had got into the slough and were in danger of drowning. As the old coach began to climb the hill, Mr. Lincoln called out, "Driver, can't you stop just a moment?" Then Mr. Lincoln jumped out, ran back, and lifted the little pigs out of the mud and water and placed them on the bank. When he returned, his companion remarked: "Now, Abe, where does selfishness come in on this little episode?" "Why, bless your soul, Ed, that was the very essence of selfishness. I should have had no peace of mind all day had I gone on and left that suffering old sow worrying over those pigs. I did it to get peace of mind, don't you see?"

We've seen in the second chapter that some of the fans of empathy are similarly cynical, seeing empathy's altruistic acts as emerging out of selfishness. If I feel your pain, then I'm in pain, and purely selfish motivation might then drive me to make your pain go away.

We've also seen that this is an unlikely explanation. If I'm in pain because I'm feeling your pain, there is a much easier way to make my pain go away than helping you—I can turn my head and stop thinking of you; the empathic connection is broken, and I'm right as rain. Then there's Batson's research, which shows that people tend to help even when escape is readily available. This is a problem for the selfishness theory of the power of empathy and is more consistent with the view that empathy motivates good behavior (when it does) by exploiting positive sentiments that are already present.

Also, with due respect to Hobbes and Lincoln, their explanations of their own behavior are question-begging. Suppose they were right that their actions were motivated by their selfish interests. This just pushes the question back. Why would Hobbes be constituted to feel good when helping another? Why would Lincoln feel bad—getting no peace of mind—if he refrained from helping when the opportunity presented itself? Even accepting their explanations as true, then, these explanations assume a nonselfish psychology that underlies these selfish desires.

Some who hold the cynical view think that they're being hard-boiled and scientific—they think that this sort of "psychological egoism" is forced upon you when you give up romantic or religious conceptions of human nature and take evolution seriously. Since the amoral force of natural selection has shaped our minds, they argue, genuinely altruistic motivations are a myth. All we really want is to survive and reproduce.

I've heard this argument too often to ignore it. But it's really a mess, wrong about natural selection and wrong about psychology.

Natural selection might be selfish (in a metaphorical sense), but if so, it's selfish about genes, not individuals. The story goes that J. B. S. Haldane was asked if he would give his life to save his brother and he said that he wouldn't, but he would happily do so for two brothers or eight cousins. Only a biologist would say something like that, but Haldane was nicely expressing how evolution works. From a genetic perspective, Haldane should care just as much about his two brothers and eight cousins as he cares for himself, because their bodies contain, on average, the same distinctive genetic material as his own body. In fact, genes that caused a person to sacrifice his life in order to save *three* brothers or *nine* cousins would have an advantage over genes that caused a person to save himself at all costs. The "goals" of natural selection transcend our bodies. So, strange as it might seem, selfish genes create altruistic animals, motivating kindness toward others.

If you choose to be selfish, then, you can't justify yourself by saying you're following the lead of your genes—caring just about yourself is profoundly *un*biological.

Then there is a confusion about psychology. The claim that we actually only care about survival and reproduction confuses the goals of natural selection (again, metaphorically speaking) with the goals of the creatures who have evolved through natural selection, including us. The difference between the two is obvious when you think about other domains. From the perspective of natural selection, the "goal" of eating is to sustain the body, to keep it going so that the genes we carry can replicate themselves. But this isn't what motivates dogs, ants, tigers, and people to eat. We eat because we're hungry, or bored, or anxious, or want to be good guests, or hate ourselves, or whatever.

There are no deep teleological musings about genetic survival running through our heads as we dig into a bag of potato chips. As William James put it, if you ask your average man why he eats, "instead of revering you as a philosopher, he will probably laugh at you for a fool."

Similarly, there is an obvious evolutionary motivation for sexual intercourse (it leads to children), but this is very different from the psychological motivations for sex, which most of the time *don't* include a desire to have children. Surely this is true for other species: When mice mate, they don't consciously intend to make more mice.

And the same considerations hold for kindness. We are naturally kind because our ancestors who were kind to others outlived and outreproduced those who didn't. But that doesn't mean that when people help others they are thinking about survival and reproduction any more than when people eat and have sex they are thinking about survival and reproduction. Rather, evolution has shaped people to be altruistic by instilling within us a genuine concern for the fate of certain other individuals, by making us compassionate and caring.

And not just people. Of course many animals—and all mammals—care for their offspring, but their helping and kindness go beyond this. Frans de Waal has done the classic work here, compiling a particularly large body of evidence about non-human primates. He finds that chimpanzees will rescue one another when they get in trouble, and sometimes act to increase others' pleasure and decrease others' pain. For instance, when a chimpanzee loses a confrontation with another and is in physical pain (and perhaps, if this isn't too much of a stretch, feeling emotional pain, possibly humiliation), often another chimpanzee will approach the loser and pat and soothe and comfort him.

The existence of these capacities in chimps suggests that you might find them in young humans as well. And toddlers do seem to care about others. Some experiments explore this by getting adults to act as if they are in pain (such as the child's mother pretending to bang her knee or an experimenter pretending to get her finger caught in a clipboard) and then seeing how children respond. It turns out that they often try to soothe the adults, making an effort to make their pain go away. Other studies find that toddlers will help adults who are struggling to pick up an object that is out of reach or struggling to open a door. The toddlers do so without any prompting from the adults, not even eye contact, and will do so at a price, walking away from an enjoyable box of toys to offer assistance. They really do seem to want to help.

But what about empathy? What are the developmental origins of feeling what others feel?

You might think we already answered the question of empathy's origin in an earlier chapter when we described its neural basis. But it's too big a jump from the fact that empathy is in a certain part of the brain to say that it's something we're born with. All our capacities reside in our brains, after all. (Where else could they be?) Reading, playing chess, and going on Facebook all light up parts of our brains, and none of them are innate. Perhaps this is true of empathy as well. In particular, some theorists have argued that brain areas involved in empathy are the product of experience with the world, not what we start off with.

Others would argue that there is evidence of empathy from the start. One of the best-known examples is from the work of Andrew Meltzoff, who found that if you stick out your tongue at a baby, the baby is likely to stick out his or her tongue back at you. This can plausibly be seen as reflecting an empathic connection between baby and adult, grounded in the baby putting him or herself in the shoes of another.

This is controversial, as some researchers are skeptical about what tongue protrusion actually shows. Perhaps, they argue, this isn't imitation at all. Perhaps babies are freaked out when an adult sticks out his tongue at them, and they stick out their own tongues in surprise! But Meltzoff and his colleagues have responded with some recent studies that do find evidence for a convergence between self and other; you find similar patterns of brain activation, for instance, between a baby getting her face stroked and a baby watching a video of another baby getting her face stroked. And certainly later on in the first year of life, the evidence for imitation gets stronger, and you see babies imitating all sorts of specific facial expressions of the adults around them.

What about empathic distress—do babies feel the pain of those around them? Charles Darwin thought so, and gave an example from his son William. He writes: "With respect to the allied feeling of sympathy"—keep in mind that *sympathy*, in the nineteenth century, meant what *empathy* means now—"this was clearly shown at six months and eleven days by his melancholy face, with the corners of his mouth well depressed, when his nurse pretended to cry."

Findings from more recent studies are consistent with Darwin's observation. Even days after birth, babies get upset by hearing other babies cry—more upset than if they hear a recording of their own crying. And there is abundant evidence that one- and two-year-olds are bothered by seeing others in pain.

In my last book, *Just Babies*, I cited all this as evidence for early empathy. But I'm no longer sure that's true. All these anecdotes and experimental findings can be readily accounted for in terms of caring for others without any sort of empathic feeling. William's sadness, for instance, might reflect the fact that he was sad that his nurse seemed to be suffering—but this doesn't entail that he was feeling her pain in any real empathic sense.

What's more decisive are reports of how older toddlers sometimes respond to the pain of others by getting upset and then soothing themselves. This really does suggest that they are in some sort of empathic distress. Interestingly, this sort of response doesn't seem limited to people, or even primates. In one study, rats were trained to press a bar to stop other rats from receiving painful electric shocks. Some of the rats didn't press the bar, but this failure to act wasn't because they were indifferent to the suffering of other members of their species; it was because they were overwhelmed by it. As the investigators put it, they "retreated to the corner of their box farthest from the distressed, squeaking, and dancing animal and crouched there, motionless."

But do these empathic reactions generate moral behavior? After all, you can respond to the suffering of others without knowing that you are responding to the suffering of others. More than once I've found myself in a dark mood and only later realized that it was because I had been interacting with someone who was depressed. (Psychologists sometimes call this "emotional contagion.") Without an appreciation of the source of one's suffering, the shared feeling is morally inert. What gives empathy its power, after all, is that we appreciate that we are feeling what another feels. If I feel your pain but don't know that it's your pain—if I think that it's *my* pain—then I'm not going to help you. If this is true for toddlers, then their kind acts cannot be driven by empathy.

We're arriving now at the central issue: Early in development, we see kindness and compassion reflected in children's soothing and helping. And early in development, though just how early is a matter of debate, we see children suffering in response to the suffering of others. So the core question is whether these two things are connected—when children help others, is it because they are feeling their pain?

Paul Harris has reviewed the literature on this topic, and he argues that the evidence for this connection isn't there. For one thing, there are several anecdotes suggesting that young children are capable of helping without showing any distress. Consider Len: "The 15-month-old, Len, was a stocky boy with a fine round tummy, and he played at this time a particular game with his parents that always made them laugh. His game was to come toward them, walking in an odd way, pulling up his T-shirt and showing his big stomach. One day his elder brother fell off the climbing frame in the garden and cried vigorously. Len watched solemnly. Then he approached his brother, pulling up his T-shirt and showing his tummy, vocalizing, and looking at his brother."

We can't rule out the possibility that Len was in some hidden empathic anguish with his elder brother. But he sure didn't act distressed, and one-year-olds are not good at hiding their feelings. If we take this story at face value, then, it looks as if Len was worried about his brother and wanted to cheer him up, but wasn't suffering himself. This is caring without empathy.

We find the same phenomenon in the research mentioned earlier in which adults pretend to be distressed in front of children. Children often respond by trying to help the person in trouble, first with simple physical acts like patting and hugging and then with more sophisticated responses like saying "You be

OK" or bringing over a toy or some other helpful object. But the children do not typically show signs of distress themselves. The only times that they reliably seem to get upset is when they themselves cause the suffering of another person, but here the negative response is most likely due to guilt and perhaps fear, not empathic engagement.

Or consider a classic study in which pairs of six-month-olds were observed as they interacted in a playroom in the presence of their mothers. Sometimes one of the babies would become distressed, and sometimes the other baby would react by touching or gesturing toward him or her. But again, there was no evidence that the distress of one baby ever bothered another baby.

We've been talking about babies and toddlers, but I'll end with an observation about chimpanzees. We've discussed the evidence for kindness in nonhuman primates and mentioned Frans de Waal's fascinating work on consolation in chimpanzees, looking at behaviors such as kissing, embracing, and gentle touching of an animal who has just lost a confrontation. These behaviors cannot be attempts at peacemaking, as they are directed toward victims, not aggressors. They really do seem to be motivated by a desire to make the victim feel better. If a human did this, you would have no hesitation in describing the actions with words like *kindness* and *compassion*.

But Paul Harris points out something interesting here. When you look at pictures of the interactions, you see the victim's face contorted in anguish, but you don't see anguish in the consolers, just concern. If it's hard to read human minds, it's *really* hard to read other species' minds, but it sure looks as if the chimps care about the creatures they are helping—but are not mirroring their feelings.

I don't think we know enough about development in either children or chimps to be entirely confident in our conclusion. It is possible that some new discoveries will come out showing that empathy is somehow necessary for morality to blossom. But right now, as best we know, empathy is not like milk.

CHAPTER 5

Violence and Cruelty

In April of 1945, in the Dachau concentration camp, several men were lined up against the wall, tortured, and shot. Such savagery was typical for Dachau. Tens of thousands of prisoners had been murdered there, through starvation, execution, the gas chamber, and even grotesque medical experiments. But this incident happened after the camp had been liberated. The victims were captured German soldiers, and it was the American liberators who were doing the killing.

Captain David Wilsey described the incident in a letter to his wife: "I saw captured SS tortured against a wall and then shot in what you Americans would call 'cold blood'—but Emily! God forgive me if I say I saw it done without a single disturbed emotion BECAUSE THEY SO HAD-IT-COMING after what I had just seen and what every minute more I have been seeing of the SS beasts' actions."

Later he wrote: "Did I 'confess' how PASSIVELY my canteen cup was used to pour icy riverwater down SSers half-naked backs as they stood for hours with a two-arm-up-Heil-Hitler before being shot in cold blood? A truly bloodthirsty (I'd never

seen it before) combat engineer from California asked to bor-
row my cup in performing his 'preliminaries' to roaring his .45
automatic right into the face of 3 SSers. He was bloodthirsty and
nothing else would have ever 'satisfied' that boy for his brother's
death at the hands of the SS."

This chapter is about violence and the intentional infliction
of suffering, including murder, rape, and torture. I lead with this
story because it illustrates the complexity of the topic. The men
who murdered the German soldiers were not sadists or psychopaths. They were driven by strong moral feelings. A few months
later, the U.S. military released an investigation of the events
at Dachau and recommended that several soldiers be court-
martialed. The charges were dismissed by General Patton, and
the incident was largely forgotten, discussed only by historians.
I imagine that some people reading this now will believe that
Patton's decision was correct, that the soldiers' behavior was ex-
cusable, perhaps even right.

There is no shortage of single-factor theories of violence
and cruelty, theories about the one critical ingredient that we
can blame for everything that goes wrong in the world. Those
that I'm most concerned about here, for obvious reasons,
implicate lack of empathy. In *The Brothers Karamazov*, Ivan
Karamazov says that without God, all things are permitted.
Some psychologists would repeat this maxim but replace *God*
with *empathy*. If they are right, it would refute the theme of
this book.

One version of this theory proposes that evil is caused by
dehumanization and objectification, by seeing people as somehow less than human, perhaps as nonhuman animals or as objects. Once we think of people in this way, it's easy to kill or

enslave or degrade them. If it's true, as some believe, that empathy blocks this dehumanization process, it would be a strong argument in its favor—empathy would save us from our worst selves.

There are other accounts of violence that don't implicate empathy directly. Some see certain violent actions as reflecting a loss of control. This is supported by the finding that alcohol and other drugs are involved in a lot of bad behavior. By one estimate, alcohol is implicated in over half of violent crimes. This impulse-failure account is consistent as well with the fact that those who commit crimes often show lack of control in other domains of their life: They're more likely to smoke, get into car crashes, have unwanted pregnancies, and so on.

From this perspective, violence is a glitch in the system, something gone wrong. Adrian Raine has likened violent crime to a kind of cancer, as both are products of a combination of genes and environment, and both can be seen as diseases that deserve treatment.

But there is another, opposite, view, popular among economists and evolutionary theorists. This is that violence is an essential part of life, an often rational solution to certain problems. Cancer is an aberration, an illness, something that could be cleanly excised from the world: If it were eradicated tomorrow, the rest of human life would remain happily intact. But violence is part of human nature, shared with other animals, evolved for punishment, defense, and predation. And unless we are transformed into angels, violence and the threat of violence are needed to rein in our worst instincts. You can have a world without cancer, but there will never be a world without violence. Since the recipients of violence are rarely pleased with the violence directed toward them, then, in the eyes of some, at least, there will never be a world without evil.

How can we best understand evil? Roy Baumeister begins his invaluable book *Evil: Inside Human Violence and Cruelty*, by saying that all his examples will come from real life. He will not discuss Iago, Hannibal Lecter, Freddie Kruger, Satan, Keyser Söze, or the Brotherhood of Evil Mutants.

For Baumeister, these fictional portrayals are worse than useless, as they tend to assume what he calls "the myth of pure evil"—the idea that evil is a mystical and terrible force, something alien to most of us. Possessed with this force, certain people are intentionally cruel, driven by malevolence, wanting suffering for its own sake. Think of how Alfred describes the Joker to Batman in *The Dark Knight*: "Some men aren't looking for anything logical, like money. They can't be bought, bullied, reasoned, or negotiated with. Some men just . . . Some men just want to watch the world burn."

The psychiatrist and serial killer Hannibal Lecter was introduced in the books of Thomas Harris and has been reimagined on television and in many movies (including *Silence of the Lambs*, where he is played by Anthony Hopkins). Hannibal, we are told over and over again, is "a monster." He kills many people, some in horrific ways (I stopped watching the television show for a while after an episode in season two, in which Hannibal captured yet another serial killer, cut off one of his legs, and forced him to consume himself). And yet Hannibal is a strangely appealing monster; he is civilized and urbane, often directing his violence toward those who we are led to believe deserve it, and he does have certain limits—no sexual assault, for instance. (It's a discussion for another day why so many of us find such a character interesting to watch; what sort of pure evil is entertaining and what isn't.)

Hannibal is presented as a creature different from the rest of us. There are many names given to such creatures. They are *monsters, animals,* or *superpredators*—the last a term that became popular in the 1990s to refer to certain violent teenagers. They are *sociopaths* and *psychopaths,* words that have their technical meanings but are commonly used simply to refer to really awful people, those who don't care about others the way the rest of us do.

We'll discuss below the claim by David Livingstone Smith that we see certain people as less than human, as lacking fundamental human traits, and that this is the source of much cruelty. But Smith also notes that one type of individual we are prone to dehumanize is the person who does evil. The Nazis dehumanized the Jews; we now dehumanize the Nazis.

The myth of pure evil has many sources. One is what Steven Pinker calls "the moralization gap"—the tendency to diminish the severity of our own acts relative to the acts of others. You can see this in reports of violent criminals who are puzzled why people are making such a big deal of their crimes. The most extreme example is Frederick Treesh, one of a group of three "spree killers," who allegedly told a police officer, "Other than the two we killed, the two we wounded, the woman we pistol-whipped, and the light bulbs we stuck in people's mouths, we didn't really hurt anybody."

In one study, Baumeister and his colleagues asked people to recall either an instance where they angered someone or one where they were angered by someone else. When people remembered incidents in which they were the perpetrator, they often described the harmful act as minor and done for good reasons. When they remembered incidents in which they were the victims, they were more likely to describe the action as significant, with long-lasting effects, and motivated by some combination of irrationality and sadism. Our own acts that upset others are innocent or forced; the acts that others do to upset us are crazy or cruel.

The finding isn't surprising if you consider that violent or harmful acts matter a lot more to the victim than to the perpetrator. If John punches Bill, the event will usually mean more to Bill than to John; both the physics and psychology of punching mean that it has more of an impact on whoever's on the receiving end. Being raped or assaulted can have a powerful effect on someone's life, but it can matter a lot less to the person who committed the rape or assault. Or, to dial it down quite a bit, certain remarks—a sarcastic reply, a curt dismissal—can often greatly hurt the recipient but be immediately forgotten by the speaker. Now there are exceptions: Some of us obsess about offenses we may have caused when the other person didn't even notice an offense. And there are stories of criminals racked with guilt about a crime they committed long after their victim has forgotten it. But when it comes to serious acts, it's almost always the case that the ramifications are worse for the victims than for the perpetrators.

The moralization gap leads to a natural escalation of reprisals, both at the everyday level—disputes among friends, siblings, spouses—and at the level of international conflict. You do something nasty to me, and this seems so much nastier (more significant, unjustified, just meaner) to me than it does to you. And when I retaliate in what I see as an appropriate and measured way, it seems disproportionate to you, and you respond accordingly, and so on. In this way, married couples say increasingly hurtful things, and the citizens of clashing nations react with shock and anger when their own tough but fair actions are met with vile atrocities. It's a wonder we don't all end up killing each other.

The moralization gap is one reason among many that we rarely see ourselves as the evil ones. As Baumeister puts it, "If we as social scientists restrict our focus to actions that everyone *including the perpetrator* agrees are evil, we will have almost nothing to study." It is surprising to see how often the worst people in the world—rapists interviewed in prison, say—see themselves as the real victims. They are wrong to see themselves as innocents, but we are wrong as well to see them as different creatures from the rest of us.

If you want to think about evil, real evil, a better way to proceed is this: Don't think about what other people have done to you; think instead about your own actions that hurt others, that made others want you to apologize and make amends. Don't think about other nations' atrocities toward your country and its allies; think instead about the actions of your country that other people rage against.

Your response might be: Well, none of *that* is evil. Sure, I did some things that I regret or that others blame me for. And yes, my country might have done ugly things to others. But these were hard choices, tough calls, or perhaps honest mistakes, never the consequence of some sort of pure malice. Precisely. This is how people typically think of their past evil acts.

I don't want to overstate this. Some evil is done by people who really are different from the rest of us. There are sadists who get pleasure from the pain of others—though they are rare, so much so that the big book of psychiatric diagnoses, *The Diag-*

nostic and Statistical Manual, doesn't even have an entry for them. No doubt there are souls so corrupted that they really do, as Alfred put it, want the world to burn. And surely there are honest-to-God psychopaths, who despite their small numbers are responsible for a relatively great amount of crime and misery. But even for many of these individuals, the idea of pure evil is a nonstarter when it comes to explaining their actions.

Indeed, some argue that the myth of pure evil gets things backward. That is, it's not that certain cruel actions are committed because the perpetrators are self-consciously and deliberatively evil. Rather it is because they think they are doing *good.* They are fueled by a strong moral sense. As Pinker puts it: "The world has far too much morality. If you added up all the homicides committed in pursuit of self-help justice, the casualties of religious and revolutionary wars, the people executed for victimless crimes and misdemeanors, and the targets of ideological genocides, they would surely outnumber the fatalities from amoral predation and conquest."

Henry Adams put this in stronger terms, with regard to Robert E. Lee: "It's always the good men who do the most harm in the world."

This might seem perverse. How can good lead to evil? One thing to keep in mind here is that we are interested in beliefs and motivations, not what's good in some objective sense. So the idea isn't that evil is good; rather, it's that evil is done by those who think they are doing good.

Tage Rai, summarizing his work in collaboration with Alan Fiske, takes this view and pushes it to the extreme, arguing that moralization is the main cause of violence and cruelty. Here is his short list of some of the bad things people do: "war, torture, genocide, honour killing, animal and human sacrifice, homicide, suicide, intimate-partner violence, rape, corporal punishment, execution, trial by combat, police brutality, hazing, castration, dueling . . ."

What do they have in common? Rai argues that such acts aren't the result of sadistic urges, self-interest, or loss of control. Rather, the best explanation relates these acts to *morality*, to "the exercise of perceived moral rights and obligations."

It shouldn't be surprising that morality can incite violence. Morality leads to action; it gets you to stick your nose in other people's business. I don't like raisins. But this isn't a moral belief, so it just means that I don't eat raisins; it doesn't motivate me to harass others who behave differently than I do toward raisins. I also don't like murder. But this *is* a moral belief, so it motivates me to try to stop others from doing this, to encourage the government to punish them, and so on. In this way, moral beliefs motivate action, including violent action.

Morality is motivating. I read a story earlier today, from many years ago, about a man who went with his wife and children to the beach in Dubai. His older daughter, a twenty-year-old, went out for a swim and started to struggle in the water and scream for help. The father was strong enough to keep two lifeguards from rescuing her. According to a police officer, "He told them that he prefers his daughter being dead than being touched by a strange man." She drowned.

Now you'd be seriously missing the point if you saw the father's action as the product of sadism, indifference, or psychopathy. It was the product of moral commitment, no different in the father's mind than if he were struggling to prevent his daughter from being raped.

One's perspective matters a lot in these cases. After the attacks on the twin towers on September 11, 2001, some Palestinians celebrated in the streets, a reaction that many Westerners took to reflect moral depravity. But when Americans celebrated after the killing of Osama bin Laden in 2011, or when Israelis hooted and cheered as bombs dropped over Gaza in 2014, the celebrants didn't think they were doing anything shameful at all.

These different perspectives on the moral nature of certain violent acts complicates things. Rai ends his interesting essay on this topic by saying: "Once everyone, everywhere, truly believes that violence is wrong, it will end." I disagree. I don't think violence will ever end. This is because I don't believe—let alone truly believe—that violence is always wrong. My moral compass sometimes tells me that violence is the right thing to do.

I believe, for instance, that people have a right to use violence—indeed that they are morally obliged to do so—to defend themselves and others from assault, and in some cases have a right to be violent toward those who would steal their stuff. (If someone snatched my last loaf of bread, I'd try to wrestle it from him.) And I wouldn't want to live in a world where the state had no power to punish those who violated the law. Certain important social interactions, like trade, involve some notion of enforcement—if I hand you a dollar for an apple, and you keep the dollar and don't hand over the apple, we all benefit from a world where I can call someone to intervene and make you give me the apple or return the dollar. If such an intervention isn't ultimately backed up with force, it's toothless, so without violence or the threat of violence, the world would fall apart.

The examples above are meant to be uncontroversial—few people believe that we shouldn't be allowed to defend ourselves from assault. Other moral claims about violence are more controversial. My own moral view says that state violence toward another nation—including war—is justifiable, even demanded, under certain circumstances, and this doesn't have to be an act of self-defense. (Even if there were no other considerations, the United States would have been right to invade Germany to liberate camps such as Dachau.) I think boxing, football, and martial arts are acceptable forms of recreation and entertainment, despite their violent nature. I think that under certain conditions the state should be allowed to forcibly stop a person from committing suicide.

My point isn't to convince you of any of this but just to note that the moral issues involving violence are complicated. It's not that there is some *mistake* that most people are making, that if only we could get everyone to realize that violence is not the answer, the world would be a much better place. We are always going to have a world with violence. We have to grapple with the difficult question of how much and what kind.

We've seen clear cases where violence and cruelty are motivated by moral views. But often this is not the case. It might be true that not many rapists, muggers, and thieves think of themselves as truly evil people—rather, they would say that they're victims of circumstance, someone else is to blame, their needs are greater than others', and so on. But few are so deluded as to see their actions as fulfilling a moral calling. The other explanations for harming others, including simple desires for money, sex, status, and so on, have to come into play as well.

And this brings us to the issue of empathy. Not everyone is

willing to make others suffer in order to achieve what he or she wants. Perhaps empathy provides the brakes. Greed makes us want to knock someone down and take their money; empathy holds us back. Anger makes us want to respond to an insult by punching someone in the face; empathy restrains us.

I told a story earlier from Jonathan Glover about a woman who lived close to a concentration camp and felt empathy for those being tortured. Her response was to ask that the torture be done elsewhere, where it wouldn't disturb her. This was one of a series of examples meant to show how empathy need not make us good. But there are also cases where empathy *does* seem to make us better, to block our worst impulses. Glover also tells a story from George Orwell, when he was fighting in the Spanish Civil War and came across a solider holding up his trousers with both hands: "I did not shoot partially because of that detail about the trousers. I had come here to shoot at 'Fascists,' but a man who is holding up his trousers isn't a 'fascist'; he is visibly a fellow creature, similar to yourself, and you don't feel like shooting at him."

I concede that empathy can serve as the brakes in certain cases. But I will argue here that it's just as often the *gas* — empathy can be what motivates conflict in the first place. When some people think about empathy, they think about kindness. I think about war.

I'm aware that this is an unusual claim. Here is a more standard perspective on the role of empathy, written by Simon Baron-Cohen as part of a response to an article that I wrote. His example is the war in Gaza, which was at its height as we were writing:

> Consider Israeli Prime Minister Benjamin Netanyahu's decision: Should I command the Israeli Defense Force to bomb

a rocket launcher that Hamas is firing from within a UN school, and in the process risk killing innocent Palestinian children?

Using the unempathic, rational cost-benefit calculation, . . . his decision is to bomb the Hamas rocket launcher.

Now imagine Netanyahu uses empathy to make his decision. Suppose he says to himself *"What would it be like* if I were the father of a Palestinian child killed by an Israeli bomb? What would it be like if that Palestinian child were my child, terrified by the bombs raining down?" Using empathy the answer would likely be to find a different way to render the whole region safe.

The same applies to the decision by the leaders of Hamas to fire a rocket at Israel, despite Israel's possession of the new Iron Dome defense system. If Hamas uses the unempathic, cost-benefit calculation, . . . [it] leads to firing the rocket at Israel.

But suppose the leaders of Hamas say to themselves, *"What would it be like if* I were the Israeli child trying to go to sleep at night, when the sirens go off?" Or, "What would it be like if that elderly Israeli woman running for the shelter were my mother?" The answer would be to find a different way to protest against injustice and inequality.

Much of this makes sense. If we were to have empathy for our enemies, it would block us from hurting them.

Unfortunately, though, this isn't how empathy works. Consider what happens when a country is about to go to war. Do leaders gain support by making rational arguments with statistical assessments of costs and benefits? Is the decision driven by the sort of "unempathic cost-benefit calculation" that Baron-Cohen complains about? Does this cold-blooded calculation explain the psychology of those who supported either side of the conflict in Gaza—or the American invasion of Iraq?

Not so much. What is more typical is that people feel deeply about the crimes done in the past toward their families or compatriots or allies. Consider how the Israeli reaction to the news of three murdered Israeli teenagers spurred the attacks on Gaza, or how Hamas and other organizations used murdered Palestinians to generate support for attacks against Israel. If you ask a proponent on either side why they are killing their enemies' children, they don't spout the sort of bureaucratic number crunching that Baron-Cohen worries about. They more often talk about the harm that's been done to those they love.

Some would argue that the solution is more empathy. For Israelis, then, empathy not just for their neighbors sitting in the café but for the suicide bomber who set off the bomb that maimed them. For the Palestinians, empathy not just for their brothers and sisters who had their homes crushed by tanks but for the soldiers driving the tanks.

This is a nice thought, perhaps, but we've seen a lot of evidence by now suggesting that this is not how empathy works. Asking people to feel as much empathy for an enemy as for their own child is like asking them to feel as much hunger for a dog turd as for an apple—it's logically possible, but it doesn't reflect the normal functioning of the human mind. Perhaps there are special individuals who are capable of loving their enemies as much as they love their families. But are world leaders, such as Benjamin Netanyahu and the men who run Hamas, the sort of transcendent individuals who can override human nature in this way? I doubt it.

Also, in this case and so many others, empathy is not sufficient to guide moral action. In the end, individuals who wish to do good have to be consequentialists at least to some degree, doing the sort of cost-benefit calculation that Baron-Cohen derides. Suppose that prior military action could have stopped Hitler from killing millions in concentration camps. I believe it would have been morally right to engage in such action even thought it surely would have led to the death of innocent people. If Baron-Cohen agrees with me here, then he too recognizes the limits of empathy and the value of cost-benefit calculation.

Indeed, sometimes the right thing to do involves allowing one's own citizens to die. In World War II, the British military had cracked the Enigma code and had advance notice of impending German attacks on Coventry. But if they prepared for the attacks, the Germans would have known the code was cracked. So Churchill's government made the hard choice to let innocent people die in order to retain a military advantage, giving them a better chance of winning the war and saving a greater number of innocent lives.

The idea that empathy can motivate violence is an old one and is thoughtfully discussed by Adam Smith: "When we see one man oppressed or injured by another, the sympathy which we feel with the distress of the sufferer seems to serve only to animate our fellow-feeling with his resentment against the offender. We are rejoiced to see him attack his adversary in his turn, and are eager and ready to assist him."

I see you injured by another, and I feel your resentment, and this animates me to join your cause. Now this way of framing things can't be completely right as a theory of why we might wish to harm wrongdoers. After all, I think that someone who tortures kittens should be punished, but this isn't because I believe that the kittens themselves wish for this punishment. The relevant question isn't "What does the victim want?" It is "What would I want, if I or someone I cared about were in the position of the victim?" Smith himself later clarifies this, saying that with regard to the victim, "we put ourselves in his situation . . . we enter, as it were, into his body, and . . . we bring home in this manner his case to our own bosoms. . . ."

When scholars think about atrocities, such as the lynchings of blacks in the American South or the Holocaust in Europe, they typically think of hatred and racial ideology and dehumanization, and they are right to do so. But empathy also plays a role. Not empathy for those who are lynched or put into the gas chambers, of course, but empathy that is sparked by stories told about innocent victims of these hated groups, about white women raped by black men or German children preyed upon by Jewish pedophiles.

Or think about contemporary anti-immigrant rhetoric. When Donald Trump campaigned in 2015, he liked to talk about Kate—he didn't use her full name, Kate Steinle, just Kate. She was murdered in San Francisco by an undocumented immigrant, and Trump wanted to make her real to his audience, to make vivid his talk of Mexican killers. Similarly, Ann Coulter's recent book, *Adios, America*, is rich with detailed descriptions of immigrant crimes, particularly rape and child rape, with chapter titles like "Why Do Hispanic Valedictorians Make the News, But Child Rapists Don't?" and headings like "Lost a friend to drugs? Thank a Mexican." Trump and Coulter use these stories to stoke our feelings for innocent victims and motivate support for policies against the immigrants who are said to prey upon these innocents.

There are many causes of violent conflict, and I wouldn't argue for a moment that empathy for the suffering of victims is more important than the rest. But it does play a role. When Hitler invaded Poland, the Germans who supported him were incensed by stories of the murder and abuse of fellow Germans by Poles. As the United States prepared to invade Iraq, the newspapers and Internet presented lurid tales of the abuses committed by Saddam Hussein and his sons. More recently, the U.S. government gained support for air strikes on Syria by emphasizing the horrors inflicted by Assad and his soldiers, including the use of chemical weapons. Should we move to an all-out war against ISIS, we will see more and more images of beheadings and be exposed to more and more stories about their atrocities.

I'm not a pacifist. I believe that the suffering of innocents can sometimes warrant military intervention, as, again, in the decision by the United States to enter World War II. But empathy tilts the scale too much in favor of violent action. It directs us to think about the benefits of war—avenging those who have suffered, rescuing those who are at further risk. In contrast, the costs of war are abstract and statistical, and a lot of these costs fall upon those we don't care about and hence don't empathize with. Once the war is under way, one can try to elicit empathy for those who have suffered, particularly those on one's own side, because now the costs have become tangible and specific. But by then, it's often too late.

There hasn't been much experimental research on how empathy can spark violence, but there is a suggestive pair of studies by Anneke Buffone and Michael Poulin that directly bears on this issue.

They first asked people to describe a time in the past year when someone they were close to was mistreated, either physically or psychologically. They asked their subjects how attached they felt to this victim and then asked them whether they aggressively confronted the person who caused this mistreatment. As predicted, the more warmly they felt toward the victim, the more aggressive they said they were, consistent with a connection between empathy and violence.

As the authors acknowledge, though, this finding can be explained in many ways. Maybe it's not compassion or kindness, let alone empathy, that's motivating the aggression, but simply closeness to the victim. So they did a second experiment that better zooms in on this.

Subjects were told about a math competition for a twenty-dollar prize between two students, described as strangers, who were currently in another room of the laboratory. They then read an essay purportedly written by one of the students, which described her financial problems—she needed to replace a car and pay for class registration. The subjects were then told that they were involved in an experiment that explored the effect of pain on performance, and to make everything random they would get to choose how much pain to administer—by choosing a dosage of hot sauce—to the student the financially needy student was competing with.

The trick here concerned how the essay purportedly written by the student ended. As in the Batson studies we talked about earlier, some of the subjects read a passage designed to elicit empathy ("I've never been this low on funds and it really scares me"), while others did not ("I've never been this low on funds, but it doesn't really bother me").

As predicted, greater amounts of hot sauce were assigned

to the competitor when the person was described as distressed. Keep in mind that this competitor didn't do anything wrong; he or she had nothing to do with the student's anxiety about money.

Interestingly, the studies by Buffone and Poulin also found that there was a greater connection between empathy and aggression in those subjects who had genes that made them more sensitive to vasopressin and oxytocin, hormones that are implicated in compassion, helping, and empathy. It's not just that certain scenarios elicit empathy and hence trigger aggression. It's that certain sorts of people are more vulnerable to being triggered in this way.

I've come up with similar findings in a series of studies done in collaboration with Yale graduate student Nick Stagnaro. We tell our subjects stories about terrible events, about journalists kidnapped in the Middle East, about child abuse in the United States. And then we ask them how best to respond to those responsible for the suffering. In the Middle East case, we give a continuum of political options, from doing nothing, to engaging in public criticism, all the way up to a military ground invasion. For the domestic version, we ask about increased penalties for the abuser, from raising their bail to making them eligible for the death penalty. Then we give people Baron-Cohen's empathy scale. This has its problems, as discussed earlier, but it should give some rough approximation of how empathic people are. Just as with the genetic study of Buffone and Poulin, we found that the more empathic people are, the more they want a harsher punishment.

Let's shift from bad acts to bad people. Moralization theory claims that some terrible acts are done by those driven by a desire to do the right thing, to be moral. But plainly, other terrible acts are done by people who are not overly concerned with morality, who are thoughtless in the pursuit of their own goals, indifferent to the pain of others. They don't value others as much as they should; perhaps they even enjoy making people suffer. Maybe they lack empathy.

As we've seen, this isn't always the case. Often people who commit terrible acts are empathic and caring in other parts of their lives. One manifestation of this, often pointed out by those who want to mock vegetarians, was the concern that many Nazis had for nonhuman animals. Hitler famously loved dogs and hated hunting, but this was nothing compared to Hermann Göring, who imposed rules restricting hunting, the shoeing of horses, and the boiling of lobsters and crabs—and mandated that those who violated these rules be sent to concentration camps! (This was the punishment that he imposed on a fisherman for cutting up a live frog for bait.) Or take Joseph Goebbels, who said, "The only real friend one has in the end is the dog. . . . The more I get to know the human species, the more I care for my Benno."

But then again, some Nazis really did seem to revel in their cruelty, and some of the atrocities done at the time of the Holocaust were done with enthusiasm and relish. I said earlier that sadists are rare, but if they do exist, they were probably overrepresented among, say, concentration camp guards. Certain individuals seem to be drawn to violent conflicts, showing up not because of ideological, religious, or political commitments, but because they enjoy torturing, raping, and killing people.

This brings us to a certain special group that needs to be reckoned with, one that often comes to mind when we talk about the pros and cons of empathy. For many, members of this group constitute the perfect refutation of everything in this book.

I am talking about psychopaths. In popular culture, the term *psychopath*—or its lesser-used synonym, *sociopath*—is used to refer to a certain kind of awful, dangerous person. There is a certain vagueness to the term. Some see psychopaths as impulsive and violent people; others see them as cold-blooded and controlled. Psychopaths are sometimes described as criminals living on the fringes of society, but it's also claimed that many CEOs and world leaders are psychopaths. As Jennifer Skeem and her colleagues note, there is a lack of consensus in the scientific literature as well. Psychopaths are sometimes described as aggressive and angry, sometimes as having dulled and superficial emotions. They can be seen as reckless and impulsive, but also as clever masterminds. They are sometimes said to attain high levels of success, and yet much of the research looks at individuals who are in prison or in psychiatric institutions.

So what does it mean to be a psychopath? There is a Psychopathy Checklist, developed by the Canadian psychologist Robert Hare. This is commonly used to make decisions about sentencing, parole, and other significant matters. A variant of the checklist, which involves self-report and doesn't need professional training to administer, is used by my colleagues who study college and university undergraduates and look at how their scores relate to phenomena like their attitudes toward sexual violence and their style of moral reasoning.

The traits that comprise the Psychopathy Checklist fall into four main categories: (1) how you deal with other people, assessing traits like grandiosity, superficial charm, and manipulativeness; (2) your emotional life, including your empathic responses, or lack thereof; (3) your lifestyle, with a focus on parasitic, impulsive, and irresponsible behaviors; and (4) your propensity for bad behavior in the past, including encounters with the criminal justice system. Then there are two additional criteria, involving sex and romance.

Psychopathy Checklist-Revised (PCL-R) Factors, Facets, and Items

FACTOR 1: INTERPERSONAL-AFFECTIVE SCALE		FACTOR 2: ANTISOCIAL SCALE	
Facet 1 Interpersonal	Facet 2 Affective	Facet 3 Lifestyle	Facet 4 Antisocial
Glibness/ superficiality charm	Lack of remorse or guilt	Need for stimulation/ proneness to	Poor behaviorial controls
Grandiose sense of self-worth	Shallow affect Callousness/lack of empathy	boredom Parasitic lifestyle	Early behaviorial problems Juvenile delinquency
Pathological lying Conning/ manipulative	Failure to accept responsibility for own actions	Lack of realistic long-term goals Impulsivity Irresponsibility	Revocation of conditional release Criminal versatility

From R. D. Hare, *Manual for the Revised Psychopathy Checklist, 2nd ed.* (Toronto: Multi-Health Systems, 2003).
Note: Two PCL-R items are not included in this factor structure: namely "promiscuous sexual behavior" and "many short-term marital relationships."

Almost all the traits that this checklist assesses are negative ones. (I say "almost" because some might protest that there's nothing wrong with promiscuity.) Someone who scored the maximum on the test would be glib, grandiose, a pathological liar, manipulative, lacking guilt or remorse, emotionally shallow, and so on. So it makes sense that this checklist has some success in picking out people with a propensity for bad behavior. If I were going on a long bus ride, I'd pay quite a premium to avoid sitting next to someone who maxed out on the Psychopathy Checklist.

But it's far from clear that there is such a thing as a certain type of person who is a psychopath. Those who score high on the Psychopathy Checklist might be worse people not because the items pick out a certain syndrome or disease, but simply because they pick out bad traits. Keep in mind also that there is no objective cutoff point for what distinguishes the psychopath from the nonpsychopath; different investigators use different cutoffs depending on the study, so it's an arbitrary decision at what point to slap on the label *psychopath*.

On the other hand, the traits are not just a hodgepodge of bad attributes: There are systematic patterns. Some have argued that there are three main components of psychopathy— disinhibition, boldness, and meanness. This last component strikes me as a strangely casual word for a psychological condition, but *meanness* does nicely capture a certain set of relevant dispositions, including "deficient empathy, disdain for and lack of close attachments with others, rebelliousness, excitement seeking, exploitativeness, and empowerment through cruelty." When people talk about psychopathy in criminals, this is the trait that they are often thinking about.

This brings us to lack of empathy, as this is seen as part of meanness and it's one of the items, or traits, on the Hare checklist: "callous/lack of empathy." Many popular treatments of psychopathy see a lack of empathy as the core deficit in psychopathy. Here it is important to go back to the distinction between cognitive empathy and emotional empathy. Many psychopaths have perfectly good cognitive empathy: They are adept at reading other people's minds. This is what enables them to be such master manipulators, such excellent con men and seducers. When people say that psychopaths lack empathy, they are saying that it's the emotional part of empathy that's absent— the suffering of others doesn't make them suffer.

So is lack of empathy the core deficit that underlies psychopathy, that makes psychopaths psychopaths? There are reasons to doubt it.

For one thing, as Jesse Prinz points out, it's not that psychopaths suffer from a *specific* empathy deficit. Rather, they might suffer from a blunting of just about all the emotions. This is one of the traits assessed by the checklist—"shallow affect"—and it was observed by Hervey Cleckley in his 1941 book that provided the initial clinical description of psychopathy: "Vexation, spite, quick and labile flashes of quasi-affection, peevish resentment, shallow moods of self-pity, puerile attitudes of vanity, and absurd and showy poses of indignation are all within his emotional scale and are freely sounded as the circumstances of life play upon him. But mature, wholehearted anger, true or consistent indignation, honest, solid grief, sustaining pride, deep joy, and genuine despair are reactions not likely to be found within this scale."

For Prinz, this raises the question of whether the nastiness of psychopaths has anything special to do with empathy, as opposed to arising from, or being associated with, an overall limited emotional life.

A different concern is raised by Jennifer Skeem and her colleagues. They note that scores on both the "callous/lack of empathy" item and the "shallow affect" item are weak predictors of future violence and crime. The Psychopathy Checklist is predictive of future bad behavior not because it assesses empathy and related sentiments but because, first, it contains items that assess criminal history and current antisocial behavior—questions about juvenile delinquency, criminal versatility, parasitic lifestyle—and, second, it contains items that have to do with lack of inhibition and poor impulse control.

This conclusion about psychopaths fits well with what we know about aggressive behavior in *non*psychopaths. As we discussed in an earlier chapter, a meta-analysis summarized the data from all studies that looked at the relationship between empathy and aggression, including verbal aggression, physical aggression, and sexual aggression. It turns out that the relationship is surprisingly low.

So here's what we can say about psychopaths and empathy: They do tend to be low in empathy. But there is no evidence that this lack of empathy is responsible for their bad behavior.

One decisive test of the low-empathy-makes-bad-people theory would be to study a group of people with low empathy but without the other problems associated with psychopathy. Such individuals might exist. People with Asperger's syndrome and autism typically have low cognitive empathy—they struggle to understand the minds of others—and have been argued to have low emotional empathy as well, though here, as with psychopaths, there is some controversy as to whether they are incapable of empathy or choose not to deploy it.

Are they monsters? They are not. Baron-Cohen points out that they show no propensity for exploitation and violence. Indeed, they often have strong moral codes. They are more often the victims of cruelty than its perpetrators.

No discussion of cruelty and violence would be complete without considering dehumanization—thinking about and treating other people as if they are less than fully human. This is the cause of much of the cruelty in the world.

Some of the most interesting thinking on this topic comes from David Livingstone Smith, who explores dehumanization from the standpoint of psychological essentialism. He draws on research suggesting that people usually think of themselves and those close to them as possessing a special human essence. But not everyone is seen this way. We might see members of certain groups as having not fully realized their essences, as primitive and childlike. We might deny them an essence altogether, seeing them as nonhuman, perhaps as objects or things. And in the worst case, we can deny them a human essence and also attribute to them a subhuman essence and hence think of them as akin to dogs or rats.

One can see dehumanization in the way many Nazis thought of the Jews, in what European colonists believed about indigenous people in the Americas, and in the attitudes of slave owners in the American South. As just one example among many, the missionary Morgan Godwin said that slave owners believed that slaves lacked humanity: He had been told "That the Negro's, though in their Figure they carry some resemblances of Manhood, yet are indeed *no Men*"; rather they are "Creatures destitute of Souls, to be ranked among Brute Beasts, and treated accordingly."

This is more than just talk; such dehumanization is reflected in the treatment of these people. Consider that during much of European history, even through the twentieth century, there were human *zoos*, where Africans were put in cages for Europeans to gawk at. And dehumanization is not merely a European vice. As the anthropologist Claude Lévi-Strauss put it, for many human groups "Humankind ceases at the border of the tribe, of the linguistic group, even sometimes of the village," so much so that these groups call themselves human but see others as creatures like "earthy monkeys" or "louse's eggs."

A search of racist websites can easily find contemporary examples of this, of blacks, Jews, Muslims, and other members of despised groups being talked about as if they were nonhuman animals, lacking deep feelings and higher intellectual powers. In laboratory studies, researchers have found that people are prone to think of members of unfamiliar or opposing groups as lacking emotions that are seen as uniquely human, such as envy and regret. We can see them as akin to savages or, at best, as children.

We're focusing here on ethnicity and race, but something related to dehumanization occurs in the domain of sex. Feminist scholars such as Andrea Dworkin, Catharine MacKinnon, and Martha Nussbaum have explored the notion of "objectification," in which the objectifier (typically a man) thinks of the target of his desire (typically a woman) as less than human. In a perceptive discussion, Martha Nussbaum suggests what objectification implies about a person, including: "Denial of autonomy . . . lacking in autonomy and self-determination; Inertness . . . lacking in agency, and perhaps also in activity; Denial of subjectivity . . . something whose experiences and feelings (if any) need not be taken into account."

My own analysis, though, is subtly different. I think that a certain class of attitudes toward women actually reflects the same attitudes that Smith talks about in the domain of race. We often see dehumanization, not objectification.

Consider the depiction of women in pornography—the focus of much of the critical discussion on objectification. It is not literally true that these women are depicted as inanimate and interchangeable objects, as lacking agency and subjective experience. Rather, the women in pornography are depicted as aroused and compliant. In at least some cases, they are depicted as purely sexual beings, just lacking certain intellectual and emotional properties we normally associate with people. The real moral issue that concerns us (or should concern us) about the depiction of women in pornography isn't that they are seen as objects, but that they are depicted as lesser individuals, as similar to stupid and submissive slaves. This establishes a parallel with the sort of cases discussed by Smith.

Dehumanization is indefensible. It's obviously mistaken to think about blacks or Jews or women as lacking critical human traits like agency and self-determination and rich emotional lives, and it is a mistake that can have terrible consequences, motivating and excusing indifference and cruelty. For some people, this is why empathy is so important. Empathy blocks dehumanization and allows us to see people as they really are. If so, this would be a powerful case in its favor.

Not surprisingly, I reject this view. I think that empathy is not needed to treat people as people; it is not an essential aspect of avoiding dehumanization.

Note first that one can be cruel without dehumanization. In fact, there is a sense in which the worst cruelties rest on *not* dehumanizing the person. To see this, consider the first chapter of Smith's book *Less Than Human*, which begins with these words: "Come on dogs. Where are all the dogs of Khan Younis? Son of a bitch! Son of a whore!"

These turn out to be taunts from a loudspeaker mounted on

an Israeli jeep, directed toward the Palestinian side of the Khan Younis refugee camp. Smith gives this as an example of how individuals in conflict portray their enemy as nonhuman animals. But it's a strange example. Sure, the Palestinians are literally described as dogs. But this taunting would be odd behavior if the Israelis actually *did* think of them as dogs because, really, what would be the point? It would be one thing if the soldiers in the jeep casually described their enemies as dogs in conversations with one another—this could be pure dehumanization—but to use the description as a taunt implies the opposite, that you believe they are people and wish to demean them.

Kate Manne makes a similar argument in her discussion of the aftermath of a police shooting in Ferguson, Missouri, where police officers screamed at protesters, "Bring it, you fucking animals, bring it!" For Manne, this can best be seen not as a failure to acknowledge the protesters' humanity, but as "a slur and a battle cry," as an "insult that depends, for its humiliating quality, on its targets' distinctively human desire to be recognized as human beings."

Manne quotes Kwame Anthony Appiah as noting that those accused of dehumanizing others often "acknowledge their victims' humanity in the very act of humiliating, stigmatizing, reviling and torturing them." You see this in the treatment of the Jews up to and including the Holocaust. While much of what happened during acts of mass killing did reflect thinking of the Jews as less than human, some of the actions prior to this—the various humiliations and degradations of Jews in the Ukraine, for instance, and the delight that people took in this—reflect an appreciation of the humanity of those who were being tormented. If you don't think of them as initially possessing dignity, where's the pleasure in degrading them?

And the same occurs in the sexual realm. Here again, there can be true dehumanization. Much of sexism involves a sincere belief that women are not fully developed humans, and there is a large body of experimental research (including some work that I've done with my colleagues) suggesting that when a man is feeling sexual desire, or is simply looking at women's bodies and not their faces, there is a tendency to think of women as less agentic, as lacking autonomy and will, as not fully human. But that's not the whole story: Some acts of rape or sexual harassment or mundane everyday sexism are carried out with a full consciousness of the target's humanity—and a corresponding desire to demean and humiliate her.

In his discussion of the importance of empathy, Simon Baron-Cohen remarks that "Treating other people as if they were objects is one of the worst things you can do to another human being." I agree—but looking at the sorts of examples described above, I don't think it's the *very* worst.

I'm framing this point as an alternative to Smith's dehumanization analysis. But in response, Smith points out that this sort of degrading treatment, while not reflecting dehumanization, might reflect a *wish* to dehumanize, a desire to bring people down to the point where they are seen, and will see themselves, as less than human. Calling people "dogs" and "animals," then, is more than just insult; it's different from saying that someone is ugly and stupid. It's an attempt to shift how these people are thought of.

In support of Smith's analysis, consider how the Nazis, transporting Jews by train to the concentration camps, denied their prisoners access to toilets. One might think of this as simply a cruel thing to do, but Primo Levi describes how it can support dehumanization: "The SS escort did not hide their amusement at the sight of men and women squatting wherever they could, on the platforms and in the middle of the tracks, and the German passengers openly expressed their disgust: people like this deserve their fate, look at how they behave. These are not Menschen, human beings, but animals, it's as clear as day."

Is lack of empathy another force that supports dehumanization? I think not. There is a big difference between actively denying someone's human traits—dehumanization—and not thinking about these human traits but instead focusing on other aspects of the person. The first is terrible; the second is not.

To elaborate on this, consider some examples. A couple is lying in bed and the woman uses her partner's stomach as a pillow. Or a man in a crowd moves behind someone to keep the sun out of his eyes. Or a host is having several people over for dinner and needs to figure how much food to order from Royal Palace and where to put the chairs around a too-small table. This can all be done without considering people's thoughts and feelings, by literally thinking of people in the same way that one would think of objects. But none of this is immoral.

Similarly, I've been arguing throughout this book that fair and moral and ultimately beneficial policies are best devised without empathy. We should decide just punishments based on a reasoned and fair analysis of what's appropriate, not through empathic engagement with the pain of victims. We should refrain from giving to a child beggar in India if we believe that our giving would lead to more suffering. None of this denies that pain and suffering exist, and none of this is dehumanization in the sense that we should worry about. It's just that we are better off focusing on some things and not others in order to achieve certain good ends. Since the ends matter, this is not cruel; it's kind.

We've seen that empathy's relationship to violence and cruelty is complicated. It's not true that those who do evil are necessarily low in empathy or that those who refrain from evil are high in empathy. We've seen how empathy can make us worse people, not merely in the sense that it leads to bad policy and can mess up certain relationships but in the stronger sense that it can actually motivate savage acts.

As we think about empathy, it's useful to compare it to anger. They have a lot in common: Both are universal responses that emerge in childhood. Both are social, mainly geared toward other people, distinguishing them from emotions such as fear and disgust, which are often elicited by inanimate beings and experiences. Most of all, they are both moral, in that they connect to judgments of right and wrong. Often empathy can motivate kind behavior toward others (I should help this person); and often anger can motivate other actions, such as punishment (I should hurt this person). And they can be related to one another. We've seen that empathy can lead to anger; the empathy one feels toward an individual can fuel anger toward those who are cruel to that individual.

There are those who think that the world would be a better place without anger. Many Buddhists see it as personally corrosive and socially harmful—"unwholesome" is the word sometimes used. Owen Flanagan once described a meeting with the Dalai Lama in which he asked the leader of the Tibetan Buddhists a great question: If it would stop the Holocaust, would you kill Hitler? "The Dalai Lama turned to consult the high lamas who were normally seated behind him, like a lion's pride. After a few minutes of whispered conversation in Tibetan with his team, the Dalai Lama turned back to our group and explained that one should kill Hitler (actually with some ceremonial fanfare, in the way, to mix cultural practices, a Samurai warrior might). It is stopping a bad, a very bad, karmic causal chain. So 'Yes, kill him. But don't be angry.'"

The Dalai Lama is conceding that a rational and caring individual is going to have to engage in, or at least support, certain acts of violence, including murder. But he sees it as a necessary evil, a last resort. If there were some way to stop that very bad karmic chain without violence, that would be better. This is not the perspective of an angry person — anger feeds off the suffering of others; an angry person wants wrongdoers to suffer.

Anger, however, does make us irrational. There are many studies showing that the extent to which we punish wrongdoers corresponds to the extent of our anger. One set of experiments got people angry by showing them certain films and then asking them to judge appropriate punishments for actions that had nothing to do with what they were watching in the films. Even here, when it made no sense, the angry subjects were more punitive.

This does sound pretty bad. Many evolutionary theorists would agree that anger is a valuable adaptation, essential for our existence as a social and cooperative species. Generous and kind behavior cannot evolve unless individuals can make it costly for those predisposed to game the system and prey on others. So we have evolved emotions, including anger, that drive us to lash out at bad actors, and this makes kindness and cooperation successful. It would be a mistake, then, to see anger simply as noise in the machine, something useless and arbitrary. On the contrary, it is one of the foundations of human kindness.

But even if this evolutionary analysis is correct, it might still be true that anger leads us astray in the here and now and we would be better off without it.

So what could someone say in favor of anger? One consideration is that if other individuals are angry, you might need to be angry too. Flanagan sadly concedes this, noting that in societies where displays of anger are approved of, an individual without anger might be at a disadvantage when it comes to resolving disputes and disagreements.

A lot of things work this way, where once there is a consensus, however irrational, it's hard to opt out. You might think it's stupid to bring wine to people's houses when they have you over for dinner, but if this is what people do, you're stuck with it. If you found yourself in a maximum security prison, you might sigh despairingly at the extreme violence of your fellow prisoners—such a waste!—but you're not allowed to opt out. As the expression goes, you can't bring a knife to a gunfight.

Jesse Prinz, in an astute commentary on an article I wrote, has a stronger defense of anger. I had made the analogy between empathy and anger and suggested that they have similar limitations. But Prinz thinks I'm too quick to dismiss the moral importance of anger:

> Righteous rage is a cornerstone of women's liberation, civil rights, and battles against tyranny. It also outperforms empathy in crucial ways: anger is highly motivating, difficult to manipulate, applicable wherever injustice is found, and easier

to insulate against bias. We fight for those who have been mistreated not because they are like us, but because we are passionate about principles. Rage can misdirect us when it comes unyoked from good reasoning, but together they are a potent pair. Reason is the rudder; rage propels us forward. Bloom recommends compassion, but the heat of healthy anger is what fuels the fight for justice.

These are valid points. If I could genetically engineer the brain of my newborn baby, I wouldn't leave anger entirely out. Along the lines of Flanagan, the emotional force of anger will help protect the child and those close to the child, particularly in a world where everyone else has anger. And along the lines of Prinz, anger can be a prod to moral behavior. Many moral heroes have been people who let themselves get angry at situations that others were indifferent about, and who used anger as a motivating force for themselves and others.

I'm not as sanguine as Prinz, though, about the merits of anger as a force for social change. When we think about what makes us most angry, it doesn't seem unbiased at all—we naturally rage about injustices toward ourselves and those we love, but it requires quite a bit of effort to feel much about injustices that don't affect us. I remember the fury that many Americans felt after the attacks of September 11. It seems clear that those atrocities that don't involve us, or that we ourselves are involved in causing, don't evoke the same strength of feeling.

So when it comes to my imaginary genetically engineered child, I would put in some anger, but not too much, and I would make sure to add plenty of intelligence, concern for others, and self-control. I would be wary of removing anger altogether, but I would ensure that it could be modified, shaped, directed, and overridden by rational deliberation; that, at most, it could be a reliable and useful servant—but never a master.

That's how we should think about empathy.

CHAPTER 6

Age of Reason

Aristotle defined man as the rational animal, but he had never heard of the Third Pounder.

In the 1980s, the restaurant chain A&W wanted to create a burger that would compete with McDonald's popular Quarter Pounder. So they created the Third Pounder, which had more beef, was less expensive, and did better in blind taste tests. It was a failure. Focus groups found that the name was the problem. Customers believed that they were being overcharged, assuming that a third of a pound of beef was less than a quarter of a pound of beef since the 3 in ⅓ is smaller than the 4 in ¼.

In some regards, this tale of mathematical dunderheadedness meshes well with the theme of this book so far. I've argued that we rely too much on gut feelings and emotional responses to guide our judgments and behaviors. Doing so isn't a mistake like a mathematical error, but it's a mistake nonetheless and leads to needless suffering. We are often irrational animals.

At the same time, though, my antiempathy argument presupposes rationality. To say "This sort of judgment is flawed" and to believe it myself and to expect you to believe it assumes a psychological capacity that *isn't* subject to the same flaws. The argument, then, is that while we are influenced by gut feelings such as empathy, we are not slaves to them. We can do better, as when we rely on cost-benefit reasoning when deciding whether to go to war, or when we recognize that a stranger's life matters just as much as the life of our child, even though we love our child and don't feel any particular warmth toward the stranger.

The idea that human nature has two opposing facets—emotion versus reason, gut feelings versus careful, rational deliberation—is the oldest and most resilient psychological theory of all. It was there in Plato, and it is now the core of the textbook account of cognitive processes, which assumes a dichotomy between "hot" and "cold" mental processes, between an intuitive "System 1" and a deliberative "System 2." This contrast is nicely captured in the title of Daniel Kahneman's bestselling book, *Thinking, Fast and Slow.*

But there are many who now think that the deliberative part—"cold cognition," System 2—is largely impotent. To argue for the centrality of deliberative reasoning is seen as philosophically naive, psychologically unsophisticated, and even politically suspect.

I recently wrote a short article in the *New York Times* summarizing research on how hard it is to appreciate what's going on in the minds of others and arguing that we're bad at what's sometimes called "cognitive empathy." I figured that people would disagree with me on this, and they did, but what surprised me was the reaction to my last sentence, which was "Our efforts should instead be put toward cultivating the ability to step back and apply an objective and fair morality."

I had thought of this as a reasonable, actually pretty drab, ending, but many commentators seized on it, asking—often with scorn—exactly what this objective and fair morality was supposed to be. Did such a thing even exist? If so, why would one expect it to be a good thing? In a similar vein, a sociology professor once wrote to me and gently told me that my emphasis on reason expressed a particularly Western white male viewpoint. He didn't use the phrase, but the gist of his polite letter was that I really should check my privilege.

This sort of response really puzzles me. There are a lot of serious arguments regarding the precise sort of morality we should have—moral philosophy is *hard*—but I think the case for an objective and fair morality is self-evident. Would one prefer a subjective and unfair morality?

I can easily accept that a fan of empathy might argue (contrary to my own position) that empathy really can be fair and objective or that empathy is a necessary part of a fair and objective morality or that, at the very least, empathy is not incompatible with a fair and objective morality. That is, one might believe that the argument running through this book is mistaken and maintain that empathy is overall a good thing for someone who wants to make wise and fair decisions. One might also believe that some partiality makes sense in a personal context—if my child and a stranger were drowning and I could save just one, I'd save my child, and I don't feel that this is the wrong choice. So the partiality of empathy and other psychological processes might be morally appropriate at least some of the time. These are concerns worth taking seriously, and I've tried to respond to them throughout this book.

But it's hard for me to take seriously the claim that public policy should be made in an unfair and subjective manner (so that, say, it's right for white politicians to create laws that favor whites over blacks). As for the sociology professor, the idea that rationality is an especially white male Western pursuit is where the extremes of postmodern ideology circle around to meet with the most retrograde views of a barroom bigot. In fact, there is no reason to believe that those who are not male and not white have any special problems with reason. And with regard to the Western part, I would refer the professor to the earlier discussion of how Buddhist theology provides some exceptionally clear insights into why empathy is overrated.

There is a different critique, though, that deserves a lot more attention. This is the concern that regardless of reason's virtues, we just aren't any good at it. An undergraduate taking an Introduction to Psychology class is likely to hear in the first lecture that Aristotle's definition of man as a rational animal is flat wrong. Rather, we are creatures of intuition, of emotion, of the gut. System 1 dominates; System 2 is, well, a distant second. This is said to have been proved by neuroscience, which finds that the emotional parts of the brain have dominion, and supported by the best work in cognitive and social psychology. Contemporary psychologists are often embarrassed about Freud, but they would agree with him about the centrality of the unconscious.

I want to end this book by responding to these sorts of arguments, making the case that we are not as stupid as many scholars think we are. Then, because everyone loves a surprise ending, I'll finish off by saying some nice things about empathy.

The first attack on reason is from neuroscience. Some believe that the material basis of mental life—the fact that it all reduces to brain processes—is incompatible with a rationalist perspective on human nature.

These are hard times for anyone who wishes to defend Cartesian dualism—the idea that our minds are somehow separate from the workings of the material world, that our thinking is not done in our brain. There is evidence from neuroscience—both regular neuroscience and its sexier children, cognitive neuroscience, affective neuroscience, and social neuroscience—making it abundantly clear that the brain really is the source of mental life. It's long been known that damage to certain brain areas can impair capacities such as moral judgment and conscious experience, and over the last few decades we've developed the technology to create pretty, multicolored fMRI maps that show the material manifestations of thought. Indeed, we're getting closer to the point where we can tell what someone is thinking—or dreaming!—through neuroimaging. Someone who wanted to hold on to Cartesian dualism would have to do a lot of wiggling around to account for all this.

Some think that the neural basis of thought entails that the only way, or the best way, to study the mind is through looking at brain processes. But this is a mistake. As an analogy, consider that everything your stomach does is ultimately a physical interaction—nobody is a dualist about the tummy. But it would be crazy to try to explain indigestion in terms of particle physics. Similarly, cars are made of atoms, but understanding how a car works requires appealing to higher-level structures such as engines, transmissions, and brakes, which is why physicists will never replace auto mechanics. Or to take a final analogy closer to psychology, you can best understand how a computer works by looking at the program it implements, not the material stuff the computer is made of.

(Also, if it were really true that the best explanations were at the lowest level, then nobody should be doing neuroscience. After all, categories such as "neuron" and "synapse" are themselves quite high-level descriptions of molecules, atoms, quarks, and so on.)

All this means that you can do psychology without studying the brain, even though the mind *is* the brain. While we're at it, one can do psychology without studying evolution, even though the brain has evolved, and one can do psychology without studying child development, even though we were all once children. Of course, a good psychologist should be receptive to evidence concerning the brain, evolution, development, and much else. But the study of psychology does not *reduce* to any of these things. There are many routes to understanding. And in particular, for a lot of what psychologists are interested in, the fact that the mind is the brain just doesn't matter.

Some would disagree with this. There are scientists and philosophers who maintain that the neural basis of mental life has a particularly radical consequence. It shows that rational deliberation and free choice must be illusions. It shows that, to use the nice phrase coined by Sam Harris, each of us is little more than "a biochemical puppet."

David Eagleman makes this argument with a series of striking examples. He tells the story of how, in 2000, an otherwise normal Virginia man started to collect child pornography and make sexual overtures toward his prepubescent stepdaughter. He was sentenced to spend time in a rehabilitation center only to be expelled for making lewd advances toward staff members and patients. The next step was prison, but the night before he was to be incarcerated, severe headaches sent him to the hospital, where doctors discovered a large tumor in his brain. After they removed it, his sexual obsessions disappeared. Months later, his interest in child pornography returned, and a scan showed that the tumor had come back. Once again it was removed, and once again his obsessions disappeared.

Other examples of biochemical puppetry abound. A pill used to treat Parkinson's disease can lead to pathological gambling; date-rape drugs can induce a robotlike compliance; sleeping pills can lead to sleep-binging and sleep-driving.

It might seem that these examples are interesting just because they are so atypical. Most of the time we are not influenced by factors out of our control. As you read this book, your actions are determined by physical law, but unless you have been drugged, have a gun to your head, or are acting under the influence of a behavior-changing brain tumor, reading it is what you have chosen to do. You have reasons for that choice, and you can decide to stop reading if you want.

Eagleman would argue that this distinction is an illusion. Tumor Man is not a bizarre anomaly; he is just a case where the determined nature of behavior is particularly obvious. Speaking more generally about the implications of psychology and neuroscience, Eagleman muses: "It is not clear how much the conscious *you*—as opposed to the genetic and neural you—gets to do any deciding at all."

I disagree. I think there are critical differences between the violent acts of a paranoid schizophrenic and a killer for hire, between Tumor Man and your more mundane sexual harasser.

Now Eagleman is surely right that the difference is *not* that the reflexive cases involve actions performed by the brain while the actual deliberative cases are performed in some other way.

It's all done by the brain. Even some otherwise sophisticated commentators get confused here. One scholar, for instance, discussing serial killers, gives a musical analogy, asking us to think about a person as akin to a conductor and the brain as the orchestra. From this perspective, a bad performance can be explained as the fault of the conductor or the orchestra or both— and it would be unfair to blame the conductor for the failure of the orchestra. Similarly, "If investigation of a miscreant reveals that his brain is broken, it is likely that brain failure was at least partly responsible for his unacceptable behavior." Blame the brain, not the person! This leads to the excuse that Michael Gazzaniga has dubbed "My brain made me do it."

I agree with Eagleman that this is the wrong way of thinking. Unless one is a Cartesian dualist (and one really shouldn't be), the mind is the brain, and there is no such thing as an immaterial conductor using the brain to accomplish his will.

Rather, I'm making the distinction in a different way. My suggestion is that cases like Tumor Man are special because they involve actions that are disengaged from the normal neural mechanisms of conscious deliberation. One way to see this is that when people in these states are brought back to normal— the tumor is removed, the drug wears off—they feel that their desires and actions were alien to them and fell outside the scope of their will. Accordingly, such individuals in their altered states are less responsive to carrots and sticks: Even the threat of imprisonment did not slow down Tumor Man, because the part of his psyche that motivated his sexual behavior was disengaged from the part of his psyche that computed the long-term consequences of his actions.

In the normal course of affairs, there isn't such a disengagement. We go through a mental process that is typically called "choice," where we think about the consequences of our actions. There is nothing magical about this. The neural basis of mental life is fully compatible with the existence of conscious deliberation and rational thought—with neural systems that analyze different options, construct logical chains of argument, reason through examples and analogies, and respond to the anticipated consequences of actions.

To see this, imagine two computers. One behaves randomly and erratically; it doesn't have a rational bone in its mechanical body. The other is a deliberating cost-benefit analyzer. Plainly, both are machines: no souls here. Yet they are as different as can be. The question that remains for the psychologist is: What kind of computer are we? Or better than that—since the answer here is plainly *both*—to what extent are we irrational things and to what extent are we reasoning things?

This is an empirical question, to be resolved through experiments and observation. Neuroscience research can be relevant here, of course, but the mere fact that we are physical beings doesn't bear on the issue one way or the other. There is nothing, then, in the claim that we are rational animals that clashes with findings of neuroscience.

So we could be rational. But many psychologists would argue that they have discovered we are not. This is the second attack on reason.

Let's start with social psychology. There are countless demonstrations of how we are influenced by factors beyond our conscious control. There are studies that purport to show that our judgments and actions are swayed by how hungry we are, what the room we are in smells like, and whether or not there is a flag in the vicinity. Thinking about Superman makes you more likely to volunteer; thinking like a professor makes you better at Trivial Pursuit; being surrounded by the color blue makes you more creative; and sitting on a rickety chair makes you think that other people's relationships are more fragile.

College students who fill out a questionnaire about their political opinions when standing next to a dispenser of hand sanitizer become, at least for a moment, more politically conservative than those standing next to an empty wall. Those who fill out a survey in a room that smells bad become more disapproving of gay men. Shoppers walking past a good-smelling bakery are more likely to make change for a stranger. Subjects favor job applicants whose résumés are presented to them on heavy clipboards. Supposedly egalitarian white people who are under time pressure are more likely to misidentify a tool as a gun after being shown a photo of a black male face. People are more likely to vote for sales taxes that will fund education when the polling place is in a school.

Many of these are short-term effects, but others are not. There is evidence, for instance, that our names influence our entire lives. Is it a coincidence that the coauthors of an article in the *British Journal of Urology* are named Dr. Splatt and Dr. Weedon? Or that another urologist is named Dick Finder? Well, probably it is. But there is some statistical evidence that someone named Larry is more likely to become a lawyer, while someone named Gary is more likely to live in Georgia—that is, the first letter of your name exerts subtle influences on your preferences.

What all these examples show is that our thoughts, actions, and desires can be influenced by factors outside our conscious control and so don't make any rational sense. The sort of chair you're sitting on has no actual bearing on the sturdiness of anyone's relationship; and the fact that my first name is Paul shouldn't have influenced my choice to become a psychologist. So if it turns out that these considerations really do determine what we think and do, it would be devastating for the position that people are rational and deliberative agents.

Many do see it as devastating in this way. Jonathan Haidt captures a certain consensus when he suggests that social psychology research should motivate us to reject the notion that we are in control of our decisions. We should instead think of the conscious self as a lawyer who, when called upon to defend the actions of a client, provides after-the-fact justifications for decisions that have already been made. We are wrong to see rationality as the dog—it's actually the tail.

Now I respect the social psychology research I just summarized—I've even done some of it myself. But I don't think it shows what many think it shows.

For one thing, many of these findings are fragile. Over the last several years, the field of social psychology has been rocked by failures of replication, where the same experiment is run by a different group of psychologists and fails to find the predicted results. The issue in "repligate" isn't academic fraud, though that sometimes does happen, and there has been one prominent case where the psychologist Diederik Stapel, who reported exactly these types of counterintuitive findings (messy environments make people discriminate more), turned out to be making up his data. But the real concern has to do with normal scientific practice in this field; there are concerns that the findings have been enhanced by repeated testing and improper statistical analyses.

I once taught a seminar in which participants could satisfy their final requirement by working together on a research project, and a group of students teamed up to extend and explore a fascinating effect involving purity and morality, one that I had written about in a previous book and that raised all sorts of interesting follow-up questions. But despite numerous attempts, they couldn't replicate the original findings—and they eventually published this failure to replicate. The atypical thing about the story isn't the failure to replicate, it's the publication. Usually the project is just abandoned, though sometimes the word gets out in an informal way—in seminars, lab meetings, conferences—that some findings are vaporware ("Oh, nobody can replicate *that one*"). Many psychologists now have an attitude that if a finding seems really implausible, just wait a while and it will go away.

Not every result from a psychology lab is like this; some are powerful and robust and easy to replicate. But even for these, there is the question of real-world relevance. *Statistically* significant doesn't mean *actually* significant. Just because something has an effect in a controlled situation doesn't mean that it's important in real life. Your impression of a résumé might be subtly affected by its being presented to you on a heavy clipboard, and this tells us something about how we draw inferences from physical experience when making social evaluations. Very interesting stuff. But this doesn't imply that your real-world judgments of job candidates have much to do with what you're holding when you make those judgments. What will actually matter much more are such boringly relevant considerations as the candidate's experience and qualifications. Your assessment of gay people might be influenced by a bad smell in the room, and this supports a certain theory of the relationship of disgust and morality—one that I was interested in and the reason my colleagues and I did the study. But it's hardly clear that this matters much when people interact with one another in the real world.

Sometimes studies really are worth their press releases. Certain effects, even when they're small, can make a practical difference. And some effects aren't small at all. An example of a powerful finding is that people eat less when their food is served on small plates. One could lose weight, then, by changing one's tableware. (There, now this book contains diet tips.)

Still, even the most robust and impressive demonstrations of unconscious or irrational processes do not in the slightest preclude the existence of conscious and rational processes. To think otherwise would be like concluding that because salt adds flavor to food, nothing else does.

This point is often missed, in part because of the sociology of our field. Everybody loves cool findings, so researchers are motivated to explore the strange and unexpected ways in which the mind works. It's striking to discover that when assigning punishment to criminals, people are influenced by factors they consciously believe to be irrelevant, such as how attractive the criminals are. This finding will get published in the top journals and might make its way into the popular press. But nobody will care if you discover that people's feelings about punishments are influenced by the severity of the crimes or the criminal's past record. This is just common sense.

As an example of this, take a study in which psychologists put baseball cards on sale on eBay with photographs depicting them held either by a dark-skinned hand or a light-skinned hand. People were willing to pay about 20 percent less if they were held by the dark hands. This provides, as the authors note, a sharp demonstration of how effects of racial bias show up in a real-world marketplace—an interesting and socially significant finding. But nobody bothers to do a study looking at whether the scarcity of the card or its quality influences how much it sells for, because it's obvious that people would take into account these perfectly reasonable considerations. Findings of racial bias shouldn't lead us to forget that more rational processes exist as well, and are deeply important.

What about certain other well-known demonstrations of human irrationality? One example here is that we often ignore base rates when making decisions. Suppose you are being tested for a fatal disease. The particular test you are given will never miss this disease—if you have it, the test will be positive. But it does have a 5 percent false-positive rate, where it says you have the disease when you actually don't—that is, for every twenty people who are fine, one of them will test positive.

You test positive. Should you worry? People tend to say yes—95 percent accuracy sounds chilling. But actually, the risk depends on the base rate, on how prevalent the disease is in the population. Suppose you know that the disease is present in one out of one thousand people. Now should you worry? What are your odds of having the disease?

People tend to say the odds remain relatively high, but actually they are only about 2 percent. To see this, imagine that 20,000 people are tested: 20 people will actually have the disease and will test positive, but the test will also yield positive results for one-twentieth of the remaining 19,980 who are healthy, which is about 1,000 people. So there will be 1,020 testing positive for the disease, only 20 of whom (about 2 percent) actually have it. It's simple math when you work it out, but it doesn't seem natural.

Or take another example: Which one is more common: words ending with *ng* or words ending with *ing*? People often say that there are more words ending with *ing* because these words come to mind more easily. But if you think about it, this has to be wrong because every word that ends with *ing* also ends with *ng*, so there have to be at least as many ending with *ng*. Here, we used how quickly something comes to mind as evidence for how likely it is. This is a good heuristic but one that can lead us astray.

As a final example, imagine that you had to rule on a custody case. Here is the information about the parents:

- Parent A is average in every way—income, health, working hours—and has a reasonably good rapport with the child and a stable social life.
- Parent B has an above-average income, is very close to the child, has an extremely active social life, travels a lot for work, and has minor health problems.

Who should be awarded custody? Who should be denied custody? There may be no right answers to these questions, but one thing is for sure: The specific framing shouldn't matter. That is, since there are two individuals, and one is awarded and the other denied, they're really the same question—if you would respond A to the question about who should be awarded custody, you should respond B to the question about who should be denied, and vice versa.

But this isn't the way people respond: They show a bias toward Parent B in both cases, for both awarding and denying. One explanation for this is that when we get a question, we tend to look for data that is relevant to precisely what is being asked. So when you are asked about awarding custody, you look for considerations that would warrant getting custody and find them in Parent B (income, closeness to child), and when you are asked about denying custody, you look for considerations that would warrant being denied custody and also find them in Parent B (social life, travel, health). And this leads to irrationality—the sort of irrationality that can make a real difference in the real world.

There are many more such demonstrations. The "heuristics and biases" literature in psychology has many famous cases, and unlike some of the social psychology findings, these are robust. They make for great examples in psychology courses and can be used to liven up a conversation, a psychologist's version of a bar trick.

The existence of these "mind bugs" should be unsurprising. Some amount of irrationality is inevitable given our physical natures. We are finite beings, so there will be some cases that we get wrong. There is an analogy here with visual illusions— vision is another biological system that has evolved to perform a complex job under certain specific circumstances, so tricky scientists can often figure out how to make the system go awry by exposing people to the sorts of images that never occur in the natural world. By the same token, people often get confused when presented with problems that are expressed in terms of statistical probabilities and abstract scenarios; we are better at reasoning about problems that are expressed in terms of frequencies of events, which is just what we would expect based on the circumstances under which our minds have evolved.

A while ago, John Macnamara pointed out that the discovery of these failures of reason reveal two very different things about our minds. Most obviously, they illustrate irrationality, how things go wrong, how we are limited. But they also illustrate how intelligent we are, how we can override our biases. After all, we know that they are mistakes! Upon reflection, we appreciate the relevance of the base rates, we acknowledge that there cannot be more *ing* words than *ng* words, and we appreciate that asking about getting custody and being refused custody are really different ways of asking about the same thing. When we hear the story about the Third Pounder, we shake our heads at how dumb people can be, we wonder if the story was made up, we laugh, and we tweet about it. It turns out that every demonstration of our irrationality is also a demonstration of how smart we are, because without our smarts we wouldn't be able to appreciate that it's a demonstration of irrationality.

Much of this book has been observing this dynamic. Just as one example among many, yes, we often favor those who are adorable more than those who are ugly. This is a fact about our minds worth knowing. But we can also recognize that this is the wrong way to make moral decisions. It's this ability to critically assess our limitations—with regard to our social behavior, our reasoning, and our morality—that makes all sorts of things possible.

I've been playing defense up to now. I've been arguing that evidence and theory from neuroscience, social psychology, and cognitive psychology don't prove our everyday irrationality. But I haven't yet made a positive case for our everyday rationality, for the role of reasoning and intelligence in our lives. I'll do this now.

Think about the most mundane activities that you engage in. When you're thirsty, you don't just squirm in your seat at the mercy of unconscious impulses and environmental inputs. You make a plan and execute it. You get up, find a glass, walk to the sink, turn on the tap. This sort of seemingly mundane planning is beyond the capacity of any computer, which is why we don't yet have robot servants. Making it through a day requires the formulation and initiation of complex, multistage plans, in a world that's unforgiving of mistakes (try driving your car on an empty tank or going to work without clothes). And the broader project of holding together relationships and managing a job or career requires extraordinary cognitive skills.

If you doubt the power of reason in everyday life, consider those who have less of it. We take care of people with intellectual disabilities and brain damage because they cannot take care of themselves. Think for a minute of how much you would give up so that you or those you love wouldn't get Alzheimer's. Think about how reliant such individuals are on the help of others. Even if one is unscathed by neurological problems, there are periods of one's life where reason is diminished, such as when we are young or when we are drunk. During these periods, individuals are blocked from making significant decisions and rightfully so.

Then there are more subtle gradients of the capacity for reason. Like many other countries, the United States has age restrictions for driving, military service, voting, and drinking, and even higher age restrictions for becoming president, all under the assumption that certain core capacities, including wisdom, take time to mature.

Now some would argue that there is a threshold effect here: Once you pass an average level, you're fine. This argument is sometimes made by academics, which, as Steven Pinker points out, is rather ironic, given that academics "are *obsessed* with intelligence. They discuss it endlessly in considering student admissions, in hiring faculty and staff, and especially in their gossip about one another." Some fields are deeply invested in the concept of genius, revering those special individuals like Albert Einstein and Paul Erdős who are of such great intelligence that everything comes easy to them.

But when it comes to intelligence, there is a law of diminishing returns. The difference between an IQ of 120 and an IQ of 100 (average) is going to be more important than the difference between 140 and 120. And once you pass a certain minimum, other capacities might be more important than intelligence. As David Brooks writes, social psychology "reminds us of the relative importance of emotion over pure reason, social connections over individual choice, character over IQ." Malcolm Gladwell, for his part, argues for the irrelevance of a high IQ. "If I had magical powers," he says, "and offered to raise your IQ by 30 points, you'd say yes—right?" But then he goes on to say that you shouldn't bother, because after you pass a certain basic threshold, IQ really doesn't make any difference.

Brooks and Gladwell are interested in the determinants of success, and their goal isn't to bash intelligence but to promote other factors. Brooks focuses on emotional and social skills and Gladwell on the role of contingent factors such as who your family is and where and when you were born. Both are right in assuming these other factors to be significant. To claim that the capacity for reasoning is centrally important to our lives isn't to claim that it is *all* that matters.

Still, IQ is critically important at any level. If you had to give a child one psychometric test to predict his or her fate in life, you couldn't go wrong with an IQ test. Scores on the test are correlated with all sorts of good things, such as steady job performance, staying out of prison, good mental health, being in stable and fulfilling relationships, and even living longer. A long time ago people said things like "IQ tests just measure how good you are at doing IQ tests," but nobody takes this seriously anymore.

A cynic might object that IQ is meaningful only because our society is obsessed with it. In the United States, after all, getting into a good university depends to a large extent on how well you do on the SAT, which is basically an IQ test. (The correlation between a person's score on the SAT and on the standard IQ test is very high.) A critic could point out that if we gave slots at top universities to candidates with red hair, we would quickly live in a world in which being a redhead correlated with high income, elevated status, and other positive outcomes . . . and then psychologists would go on about how important it is to have red hair.

But the relationship between IQ and success is hardly arbitrary, and it's no accident that universities take the tests so seriously. They reveal abilities such as mental speed and the capacity for abstract thought, and it's not hard to see how these abilities aid intellectual pursuits, how they are good traits to have, and how they can have broader consequences in one's life.

Indeed, high intelligence is not only related to success; it's also related to good behavior. Highly intelligent people commit fewer violent crimes (holding other things, such as income, constant), and the difference in IQ between people in prison and those in the outside world is not a subtle one. There is also evidence that highly intelligent people are more cooperative, perhaps because intelligence allows one to appreciate the benefits of long-term coordination and to consider the perspectives of others.

It's important to emphasize that this is an "on average" thing. Certainly intellectual giftedness is no guarantee of good behavior. Eric Schwitzgebel and Joshua Rust have done a series of impressive (and entertaining) studies finding that professional moral philosophers, the people who think about right and wrong more than just about anyone else, are no better morally than other academics, at least in their everyday lives. They don't call their mothers more, they don't give more to charity, they are not more likely to return library books, and so on.

And there really are evil geniuses. When someone has evil on his or her mind, intelligence can be a valuable tool, and a dangerous one. This is a point I've made earlier regarding social intelligence—or cognitive empathy, if you want—but one can make it again regarding smarts in general. Intelligence is an instrument that can be used to achieve certain ends. If these ends are positive ones, as they are for most of us, more intelligence can make you a better person. But goodness requires some motivation; you have to care about others and value their fates.

Reason and rationality, then, are not sufficient for being a good and capable person. But my argument is that they are necessary, and on average, the more the better.

It's not just intelligence, however. I said that if you were curious about what sort of person a child would grow up to be, an intelligence test would be a great measure. But there's something even better. Self-control can be seen as the purest embodiment of rationality in that it reflects the working of a brain system (embedded in the frontal lobe, the part of the brain that lies behind the forehead) that restrains our impulsive, irrational, or emotive desires. In a series of classic studies, Walter Mischel investigated whether children could refrain from eating one marshmallow now to get two later. He found that the children who waited for two marshmallows did better in school and on their SATs as adolescents and ended up with better mental health, relationship quality, and income as adults. We've seen from studies of psychopaths that violent criminal behavior is associated with low self-control; it's interesting as well that studies of exceptional altruists, such as those who donate their kidneys to strangers, find that they have unusually high self-control.

Steven Pinker has argued that just as a high level of self-control benefits individuals, cultural values that prize self-control are good for a society. Europe, he writes, witnessed a thirtyfold drop in its homicide rate between the medieval and modern periods, and this, he argues, had much to do with the change from a culture of honor to a culture of dignity, which prizes restraint.

Once again, none of this is to deny the importance of traits such as compassion and kindness. We want to nurture these traits in our children and work to establish a culture that prizes and rewards them. But they are not enough. To make the world a better place, we would also want to bless people with more smarts and more self-control. These are central to leading a successful and happy life—and a good and moral one.

This is not a novel insight. It's been *pages* since I cited Adam Smith's *Theory of Moral Sentiments*, so consider a section where Smith discusses the qualities that are most useful to a person. There are two, and neither of them directly has to do with feelings or sentiments, moral or otherwise. Those are "superior reason and understanding" and "self-command."

The first is important because it enables us to appreciate the consequences of our actions in the future: You can't act to make the world better if you aren't smart enough to know which action will achieve that goal. The second—which we would now call *self-control*—is critical as well, as it allows us to abstain from our immediate appetites to focus on long-term consequences.

There are areas of life where we certainly seem stupid. Take politics. Social psychologists often use political irrationality as an illustration of our broader psychological limitations.

The case for political irrationality seems pretty strong. For one thing, politics is associated with certain weird factual beliefs, such as the view that Barack Obama was born in Kenya or that George Bush was directly complicit in the 9/11 attacks. My wife recently saw a Facebook post by a high school friend, warning that the president was going to remove "In God We Trust" from all paper money, a claim originally posted in a satirical online magazine, which was uncritically accepted by this person and many of her friends. This is not an isolated incident.

Rationality in political domains often does seem to be in short supply. One striking example of this is a series of studies run by Geoffrey Cohen. Subjects were told about a proposed welfare program, which was described as being endorsed by either Republicans or Democrats, and were asked whether they approved of it. Some subjects were told about an extremely generous program, others about an extremely stingy program, but this made little difference. What mattered was which party was said to support the program: Democrats approved of the Democratic program; Republicans, the Republican program. Subjects were unaware of their bias: When asked to justify their decision, they insisted that party considerations were irrelevant; they felt they were responding to the program's objective merits.

Other studies have found that when people are called upon to justify their political positions, even those that they feel strongly about, many are flummoxed. For instance, many people who claim to believe deeply in cap and trade or a flat tax have little idea what these policies actually entail.

This sure does look stupid. But there is another way to think about these findings. Yes, certain political attitudes and beliefs might not be the products of careful reasoning, but perhaps they're not supposed to be. Think about sports fans. When people root for the Red Sox or the Yankees, it's not an exercise in rational deliberation, nor should it be. Rather, people are expressing loyalty to their team. Perhaps people's views on health care, global warming, and the like should be viewed in a similar light, not as articulated conclusions, but rather as "Yay, team!" and "Boo, the other guys!" To complain that someone's views on global warming aren't grounded in the facts, then, is to miss the point. It would be like complaining that a Red Sox fan's love of her team doesn't reflect a realistic appraisal of the Sox's performance in the last few seasons.

Political views share an interesting property with views about sports teams — *they don't really matter*. If I have the wrong theory of how to make scrambled eggs, they will come out too dry; if I have the wrong everyday morality, I will hurt those I love. But suppose I think that the leader of the opposing party has sex with pigs, or has thoroughly botched the arms deal with Iran. Unless I'm a member of a tiny powerful community, my beliefs have no effect on the world. This is certainly true as well for my views about the flat tax, global warming, and evolution. They don't have to be grounded in truth, because the truth value doesn't have any effect on my life.

I am unhappy making this argument, because my own moral commitments lean me toward the perspective that it's important to try to be right about issues even if they don't matter in a practical sense. I would be horrified if one of my sons thought that our ancestors rode dinosaurs, even though I can't think of a view that matters less for everyday life. I would feel similarly if he supported ridiculous claims as true just because they fit his political ideology. We should try to believe true things.

But that's just me. Others see things differently. My point here is just that the failure of people to attend to data in the political domain does not reflect a limitation in their capacity for reason. It reflects how most people make sense of politics. They don't care about truth because, for them, it's not really about truth.

We do much better, after all, when the stakes become high, when being rational really matters. If our thought processes in the political realm reflected how our minds generally work, we wouldn't even make it out of bed each morning. So if you're curious about people's capacity for reasoning, don't look at cases where being right doesn't matter and where it's all about affiliation. Rather, look at how people cope in everyday life. Look at the discussions that adults have over whether to buy a house, what jobs to take, where to send their kids to school, what they should do about an elderly parent. Look at the social negotiations that occur among friends deciding where to go for dinner, planning a hike, figuring out how to help someone who just had a baby. Or even look at a different sort of politics— the type of politics where individuals might actually make a difference, such as a town hall meeting where people discuss zoning regulations and where to put a stop sign.

My own experience is that the level of rational discourse here is high. People know that they are involved in real decision processes, so they work to exercise their rational capacities: They make arguments, express ideas, and are receptive to the ideas of others. They sometimes even change their minds.

Let's consider again the effective altruists. Peter Singer points out that when some of these altruists talk about why they act as they do, they use language more suggestive of rational thought than of strong feelings or emotional impulse. We saw that Zell Kravinsky, for example, said that the reason many people didn't understand his desire to donate a kidney is that "they don't understand math." Another effective altruist wrote, "Numbers turned me into an altruist. When I learned that I could spend my exorbitant monthly gym membership (I don't even want to tell you how much it cost) on curing blindness instead, the only thought I had was, 'Why haven't I been doing this all along?'"

The effective altruists are unusual people, but the capacity to engage in such reasoning exists in all of us. Social psychologists are correct that some moral intuitions are impossible to justify. But as I argue in my book *Just Babies,* these are the exceptions. People are not at a loss when asked why drunk driving is wrong, or why a company shouldn't pay a woman less than a man for the same job, or why you should hold the door open for someone on crutches. We can easily justify these views by referring to fundamental concerns about harm, equity, and kindness.

Moreover, when faced with more difficult problems, we think about them—we mull, deliberate, argue. This is manifest in the discussions we have with friends and families over the moral issues that arise in everyday life. Is it right to cross a picket line? Should I give money to the homeless man in front of the bookstore? Was it appropriate for our friend to start dating so soon after her husband died? What do I do about the colleague who is apparently not intending to pay me back the money she owes me?

I've argued elsewhere that this capacity for moral reason has had dramatic consequences. As scholars like Steven Pinker, Robert Wright, and Peter Singer have noted, our moral circle has expanded over history: Our attitudes about the rights of women, homosexuals, and racial minorities have all shifted toward inclusiveness. Most recently, there has been a profound difference in how people in my own community treat trans individuals—we are watching moral progress happen in real time.

But this is not because our hearts have opened up over the course of history. We are not more empathic than our great-grandparents. We really don't think of humanity as our family and we never will. Rather, our concern for others reflects a more abstract appreciation that regardless of our feelings, their lives have the same value as the lives of those we love. Steven Pinker put this nicely:

The Old Testament tells us to love our neighbors, the New Testament to love our enemies. The moral rationale seems to be: Love your neighbors and enemies; that way you won't kill them. But frankly, I don't love my neighbors, to say nothing of my enemies. Better, then, is the following idea: Don't kill your neighbors or enemies, even if you don't love them. . . . What really has expanded is not so much a circle of empathy as a circle of rights—a commitment that other living things, no matter how distant or dissimilar, be safe from harm and exploitation.

And Adam Smith put it even better. He asks why we would ever care about strangers when our own affairs feel so much more important, and his answer is this: "It is not the soft power of humanity, it is not that feeble spark of benevolence which Nature has lighted up in the human heart, that is thus capable of counteracting the strongest impulses of self-love. It is a stronger power, a more forcible motive, which exerts itself upon such occasions. It is reason, principle, conscience, the inhabitant of the breast, the man within, the great judge and arbiter of our conduct."

As this book comes to an end, I worry that I have given the impression that I'm against empathy.

Well, I am—but only in the moral domain. And even here I don't deny that empathy can sometimes have good results. As I conceded from the start, empathy can motivate kindness to individuals that makes the world better. Even when empathy motivates violence and war, it might be a good thing—there are worse things than violence and war; sometimes the reprisal motivated by empathy makes the world a better place. The concern about empathy is not that its consequences are always bad, then. It's that its negatives outweigh its positives—and that there are better alternatives.

Also, there is more to life than morality.

Empathy can be an immense source of pleasure. Most obviously, we feel joy at the joy of others. I've noted elsewhere that here lies one of the joys of having children: You can have experiences that you've long become used to—eating ice cream, watching Hitchcock movies, riding a roller coaster—for the first time all over again. Empathy amplifies the pleasures of friendship and community, of sports and games, and of sex and romance. And it's not just empathy for positive feelings that engages us. There is a fascination we have with seeing the world through the eyes of another, even when the other is suffering. Most of us are intensely curious about the lives of other people and find the act of trying to simulate these lives to be engaging and transformative.

There is much to be said about our appetite for empathic engagement and about the appeal of stories more generally. But that would be a topic for another book.

Acknowledgments

I've been struggling with these issues since at least 2001, when my student David Pizarro and I wrote a brief article exploring the relationship between reason and emotion in moral decision-making. But I didn't think specifically about empathy until a decade later, at a conference at New York University. After the talks were over, there was a public discussion, and the philosopher Jesse Prinz made the argument that empathy is a poor moral guide; we're better off without it. I thought this was nuts and told him so. Plainly, I've reconsidered.

Over the last few years, I've developed my views on empathy in a series of articles for the general public. My first thanks go out to a series of superb editors who gave me these opportunities, including Henry Finder (*The New Yorker*), Deborah Chasman (*Boston Review*), Scott Stossel and Ross Andersen (*The Atlantic*), and Peter Catapano (*New York Times*). I have also benefited from discussions with scholarly audiences, and I am particularly grateful to Sarah-Jane Leslie for setting up a weeklong visit to the Princeton philosophy department, and to Elaine Scarry for inviting me to the Harvard Humanities Seminar. I also learned a lot from participating in an enjoyable series of online discussions with Sam Harris and from multiple visits to the *Very Bad Wizards* podcast, where I argued about empathy with my good friends David Pizarro and Tamler Sommers.

When it was time to turn my attack on empathy into a book, my extraordinary agent, Katinka Matson, made it happen. My first editor, Hilary Redmon, believed in this project, and I was saddened when she left HarperCollins to another publishing house. Denise Oswald then took over and has been as supportive, enthusiastic, and wise an editor as one could ever wish for.

I went over a draft of the book with the undergraduates, graduate students, and postdoctoral fellows of my lab, and benefited from their constructive suggestions and incisive comments. (I'll add that when you write a book that's against empathy, you open yourself up to a fair amount of jokes and teasing. My students have not resisted the temptation.) I thank Adam Bear, Joanna Demaree-Cotton, Ashley Jordan, Jillian Jordan, Matthew Jordan (all of these Jordans, none of them related—weird, right?), Kelsey Kelly, Gordon Kraft-Todd, Julia Marshall, Nick Stagnaro, and Nina Strohminger. I am especially grateful—*big shout-out*, as the kids would say—to Mark Sheskin and Christina Starmans, who went through the whole book and provided detailed comments.

Then there's everyone else. It's dazzling how much I don't know, and how willing people were to lend a hand. I approached friends, colleagues, and often strangers with questions about psychopathy, affective neuroscience, feminist philosophy, Buddhism, medical school training, political psychology, and much else. With apologies for anyone I'm forgetting, I am grateful to: Dorsa Amir, Arielle Baskin-Sommers, Daniel Batson, Daryl

Cameron, Mary Daly, José Duarte, Brian Earp, Owen Flanagan, Michael Frazier, Deborah Fried, Andrew Gelman, Tamar Gendler, Adam Glick, Jonathan Haidt, Paul Harris, Sam Harris, Gregory Hickok, Leslie Jamison, John Jost, Frank Keil, Rachel Klayman, Sara Konrath, Marianne LaFrance, Joshua Landy, Scott Lilienfeld, Larissa MacFarquhar, Megan Mangum, Kate Manne, Abigail Marsh, William Meadow, Gregory Murphy, Laurie Paul, Steven Pinker, David Pizarro, Jesse Prinz, Matthieu Ricard, Elaine Scarry, Peter Singer, Paul Slovic, David Livingstone Smith, Elliot Sober, Tamler Sommers, Jason Stanley, Jason Wright, Robert Wright, and Jamil Zaki.

As things were wrapping up, I benefited from Brenda Woodward's excellent copyediting.

I'll end with family. I am lucky enough to have a large network of relatives, blood and otherwise, who are endlessly supportive and keep me from taking myself too seriously. I'm particularly grateful to one of the smartest and kindest people I know—my mother-in-law, Lucy Wynn.

Three of my last books were about child development, and they included stories about my sons, Max and Zachary, as babies and toddlers—their first words, what disgusted them, their artwork, their moral judgments and moral actions. As they grew up, they came to have a different sort of influence on my work, providing ideas for studies, proposing clever theories, and being perfect intellectual sparring partners. While I was writing this book, they each entered the whiskey-and-cigar stage of intellectual discourse. Given their intense interest in morality and politics, we had a lot to talk about, and our conversations have had a profound influence on my views.

My wife, Karen Wynn, did *not* carefully edit multiple drafts of this book. She didn't shush the servants as I tapped away in my study; she didn't soothe my fevered brow while I worked on the endnotes. That's not our thing. What she did instead was make my life complete, filling the years in which I wrote this book with adventure, companionship, and love. Karen is restless and vivacious and brilliant, and I'm lucky to have her as my partner in life. I'd dedicate this book to her but I already promised my sister.

Notes

Prologue

4   "learn to stand"   Barack Obama, Remarks by President Obama in Address to the United Nations General Assembly, New York, September 21, 2011. Retrieved from Mark Memmott, "Obama Urges Israel, Palestinians to 'Stand in Each Other's Shoes,'" Two-Way Breaking News from NPR, September 21, 2011, http://www.npr.org/sections/thetwo-way/2011/09/21/140663207/live-blog-obama-addresses-un-general-assembly.

6   As Frans de Waal puts it   Frans De Waal, *The Age of Empathy: Nature's Lessons for a Kinder Society* (New York: Broadway Books, 2010).

As Jonathan Haidt argues   Jonathan Haidt, "The Emotional Dog and Its Rational Tail: A Social Intuitionist Approach to Moral Judgment," *Psychological Review* 108 (2001): 814–34. For a more recent exploration of these views, see Jonathan Haidt, *The Righteous Mind: Why Good People Are Divided by Politics and Religion* (New York: Vintage Books, 2012).

"We celebrate rationality"   Frans De Waal, *Primates and Philosophers: How Morality Evolved* (Princeton, NJ: Princeton University Press, 2009), 56.

In fact, my last book   Paul Bloom, *Just Babies: The Origins of Good and Evil* (New York: Crown Publishers, 2013).

7   **damage to parts of the brain**   For a classic discussion, see Antonio R. Damasio, *Descartes' Error* (New York: Random House, 2006).

    recent studies by my colleague   For example, David G. Rand, Joshua D. Greene, and Martin A. Nowak, "Spontaneous Giving and Calculated Greed," *Nature* 489 (2012): 427–30.

12 **"Your haters are your"**   Fredrik deBoer, "the future, Mr. Gittes!" May 10, 2015, http://fredrikdeboer.com/2015/05/10/the-future-mr-gittes.

Chapter 1: Other People's Shoes

16 **Robert Jay Lifton . . . talks**   Robert Jay Lifton, *The Nazi Doctors: Medical Killing and the Psychology of Genocide* (New York: Basic Books, 2000).

    nine different meanings   C. Daniel Batson, *Altruism in Humans* (New York: Oxford University Press, 2011).

    "from yawning contagion"   Jean Decety and Jason M. Cowell, "Friends or Foes: Is Empathy Necessary for Moral Behavior?" *Perspectives on Psychological Science* 9 (2014): 525.

    "nearly as many definitions"   Frederique De Vignemont and Tania Singer, "The Empathic Brain: How, When and Why?" *Trends in Cognitive Sciences* 10 (2006): 435.

    "place ourselves in his situation"   Adam Smith, *The Theory of Moral Sentiments* (Lawrence, KS: Digireads.com, 2010), 9.

17 **"persons of delicate fibres"**   Ibid., 10.

    "My grandmother would have"   John Updike, *Getting the Words Out* (Northridge, CA: Lord John Press, 1988), 17.

    "empathy kicks"   Nicholas Epley, *Mindwise: Why We Misunderstand What Others Think, Believe, Feel, and Want* (New York: Vintage Books, 2014), 44.

18 **"to see the world"**   Barack Obama, Xavier University Commencement Address, New Orleans, Louisiana, August 11, 2006, http://obamaspeeches.com/087-Xavier-University-Commencement-Address-Obama-Speech.htm.

    "Here is a sample"   Steven Pinker, *The Better Angels of Our Nature: Why Violence Has Declined* (New York: Penguin Books, 2011), 571–72.

19 everything Barack Obama has said *Center for Building a Culture of Empathy*, http://cultureofempathy.com/Obama/VideoClips.htm.

20 "Behind every progressive policy" George Lakoff, *The Political Mind: A Cognitive Scientist's Guide to Your Brain and Its Politics* (New York: Penguin Books, 2008), 47.

"leap to global empathic" Jeremy Rifkin, "'The Empathic Civilization': Rethinking Human Nature in the Biosphere Era," Huffington Post, March 18, 2010, http://www.huffingtonpost.com/jeremy-rifkin/the-empathic-civilization_b_416589.html.

"Can we reach biosphere consciousness" Jeremy Rifkin, *The Empathic Civilization: The Race to Global Consciousness in a World in Crisis* (New York: Penguin Books, 2009), 616.

"The scariest aspect" Emily Bazelon, *Sticks and Stones: Defeating the Culture of Bullying and Rediscovering the Power of Character and Empathy* (New York: Random House, 2013), 55.

"a crisis of empathy" Andrew Solomon, *Far from the Tree: Parents, Children and the Search for Identity* (New York: Simon and Schuster, 2012), 6.

21 "empathy erosion" Simon Baron-Cohen, *The Science of Evil: On Empathy and the Origins of Cruelty* (New York: Basic Books, 2012), 6.

"I do not ask" Walt Whitman, *The Complete Poems* (New York: Penguin Classics, 2004), 102.

22 these empathic prompts occur Martin L. Hoffman, *Empathy and Moral Development: Implications for Caring and Justice* (New York: Cambridge University Press, 2001).

as Jesse Prinz and others Jesse Prinz, "Is Empathy Necessary for Morality," in *Empathy: Philosophical and Psychological Perspectives*, eds. Amy Coplan and Peter Goldie (New York: Oxford University Press, 2011).

24 "'empathetic correctness'" Karen Swallow Prior, "'Empathetically Correct' Is the New Politically Correct," *The Atlantic*, May 2014. http://www.theatlantic.com/education/archive/2014/05/empathetically-correct-is-the-new-politically-correct/371442.

arguments against trigger warnings Greg Lukianoff and Jonathan Haidt, "The Coddling of the American Mind," *The Atlantic*,

September 2015, 42–53, http://www.theatlantic.com/magazine/archive
/2015/09/the-coddling-of-the-american-mind/399356.

25 **Batson and his colleagues** C. Daniel Batson et al., "Immorality from
Empathy-Induced Altruism: When Compassion and Justice Conflict,"
Journal of Personality and Social Psychology 68 (1995): 1042–54.

Leslie Jamison, author of Jeffery Gleaves, "Six Questions: *The Empathy Exams: Essays,* Leslie Jamison on Empathy in Craft and in Life,"
Harpers, March 28, 2014, http://harpers.org/blog/2014/03/the-empathy-
exams-essays.

26 **"Kravinsky is a brilliant man"** Peter Singer, *The Most Good You Can
Do* (New Haven, CT: Yale University Press, 2016), 14.

28 **"a brave comrade"** Amy Willis, "Adolf Hitler 'Nearly Drowned as a
Child,'" *Telegraph,* January 6, 2012. Thanks to Dorsa Amir for pointing
this out to me.

29 **the gap between consequentialism** For an ambitious attempt to rec-
oncile different moral theories, see Derek Parfit, *On What Matters* (New
York: Oxford University Press, 2011).

32 **toll from these mass shootings** For a detailed analysis of the statistics of mass shootings in America, see Mark Follman, Gavin Aronsen,
and Deanna Pan, "US Mass Shootings, 1982–2016: Data from Mother
Jones' Investigation," December 28, 2012, http://www.motherjones
.com/politics/2012/12/mass-shootings-mother-jones-full-data.

The town was inundated Kristen V. Brown, "Teddy Bears and
Toys Inundate Newtown," *Connecticut Post,* December 17, 2012,
http://www.ctpost.com/local/article/Teddy-bears-and-toys-inundate-
Newtown-4150578.php.

33 **"Nothing to it"** Annie Dillard, *For the Time Being* (New York: Vintage
Books: 2010), 45.

35 **Yet the program may have** For a study of the consequences of the
Massachusetts furlough program, see Massachusetts Department of
Correction, "The Massachusetts Furlough Program," May 1987, http://
www.prisonpolicy.org/scans/MADOC/Furloughpositionpaper.pdf.

37 **many legal decisions turn on** Thomas Colby, "In Defense of Judicial
Empathy," *Minnesota Law Review* 96 (2012): 1944–2015.

37 **Or take bullies** Jon Sutton, Peter K. Smith, and John Swettenham, "Bullying and 'Theory of Mind': A Critique of the 'Social Skills Deficit' View of Anti-social Behaviour," *Social Development* 8 (1999): 117–27.

38 **"'You are afraid' . . . 'Do you remember'"** George Orwell, *1984* (New York: Signet Classics, 1950), 257 and 271.

43 **"We can't feel compassion"** Lynn E. O'Connor and Jack W. Berry, "Forum: Against Empathy," *Boston Review*, August 2014, http://bostonre view.net/forum/against-empathy/lynn-e-oconnor-jack-w-berry-response- against-empathy-oconnor.

    "affective empathy is a precursor" Leonardo Christov-Moore and Marco Iacoboni, "Forum: Against Empathy," *Boston Review*, August 2014, https://bostonreview.net/forum/against-empathy/leonardo- christov-moore-marco-iacoboni-response-against-empathy-iacoboni.

44 **"Reason," David Hume famously** David Hume, *A Treatise of Human Nature* (Oxford: Oxford University Press, 1978), 415.

    "it is not that feeble spark" Adam Smith, *The Theory of Moral Sentiments* (Lawrence, KS: Digireads.com, 2010), 95.

45 **article by Peter Singer** Peter Singer, "Famine, Affluence, and Morality," *Philosophy and Public Affairs* 1 (1972): 229–43.

46 **"Nobody would buy a soda"** Larissa MacFarquhar, *Strangers Drowning: Grappling with Impossible Idealism, Drastic Choices, and the Overpowering Urge to Help* (New York: Penguin Press: 2015), 44.

47 **study by Abigail Marsh** Abigail A. Marsh et al., "Neural and Cognitive Characteristics of Extraordinary Altruists," *Proceedings of the National Academy of Sciences* 111 (2014): 15036–41.

48 **"For every *Uncle Tom's Cabin*"** Joshua Landy, "Slight Expectations: Literature in (a) Crisis" (unpublished manuscript, Stanford University, n.d.).

49 **"The good news is"** Ibid.

51 **Michael Lynch defines reason** Michael P. Lynch, *In Praise of Reason: Why Rationality Matters for Democracy* (Cambridge, MA: MIT Press, 2012).

52 **"morality is, at the very least"** James Rachels and Stuart Rachels, *The Elements of Moral Philosophy* (New York: McGraw Hill, 1993), 19.

Chapter 2: The Anatomy of Empathy

57 **people are nicer** For example, Kevin J. Haley and Daniel M.T. Fessler, "Nobody's Watching? Subtle Cues Affect Generosity in an Anonymous Economic Game," *Evolution and Human Behavior* 26 (2005): 245–56; Melissa Bateson, Daniel Nettle, and Gilbert Roberts, "Cues of Being Watched Enhance Cooperation in a Real-World Setting," *Biology Letters* 2 (2006): 412–14.

58 **Even for children** For a review, see Joseph Henrich and Natalie Henrich, *Why Humans Cooperate: A Cultural and Evolutionary Explanation* (New York: Oxford University Press, 2007).

In a typical study, Batson For a review, see C. Daniel Batson, *Altruism in Humans* (New York: Oxford University Press, 2011).

60 **The question I dread most** The discussion here is adopted from my online article "Where Does It Happen in the Brain?" EDGE Conversations, "What's the Question About Your Field That You Dread Being Asked?" March 28, 2013, https://edge.org/conversation/whats-the-question-about-your-field-that-you-dread-being-asked.

61 **"an empathy circuit"** Simon Baron-Cohen, *The Science of Evil: On Empathy and the Origins of Cruelty* (New York: Basic Books, 2012), 40.

62 **lab of Giacomo Rizzolatti** The first report of this research was Giuseppe Di Pellegrino et al., "Understanding Motor Events: A Neurophysiological Study," *Experimental Brain Research* 91 (1992): 176–80; the first article in which the term *mirror neuron* was used was Vittorio Gallese et al., "Action Recognition in the Premotor Cortex," *Brain* 119 (1996): 593–609. For a general discussion and review, see Marco Iacoboni, *Mirroring People: The New Science of How We Connect with Others* (New York: Macmillan, 2009).

63 **what DNA did** V. S. Ramachandran, "Mirror Neurons and Imitation Learning as the Driving Force behind 'The Great Leap Forward' in Human Evolution," June 1, 2000, Edge Video, transcript at https://www.edge.org/3rd_culture/ramachandran/ramachandran_index.html.

"tiny miracles" Iacoboni, *Mirroring People*, 4.

64 **Gregory Hickok notes** Gregory Hickok, *The Myth of Mirror Neurons: The Real Neuroscience of Communication and Cognition* (New York: W. W. Norton, 2014).

64 **they have been overhyped** In addition to Hickok's book, see Steven Pinker, *The Better Angels of Our Nature: Why Violence Has Declined* (New York: Penguin Books, 2011); Alison Gopnik, "Cells That Read Minds? What the Myth of Mirror Neurons Gets Wrong About the Human Brain," Slate, April 26, 2007, www.slate.com/articles/life/brains/2007/04/cells_that_read_minds.html; Richard Cook et al., "Mirror Neurons: From Origin to Function," *Behavioral and Brain Sciences* 37 (2014): 177–92.

the more general finding For a review, see Jamil Zaki and Kevin Ochsner, "The Cognitive Neuroscience of Sharing and Understanding Others' Emotions," in *Empathy: From Bench to Bedside*, ed. Jean Decety (Cambridge, MA: MIT Press, 2012).

Most of the research For reviews, see Jean Decety and Jason M. Cowell, "Friends or Foes: Is Empathy Necessary for Moral Behavior?" *Perspectives on Psychological Science* 9 (2014): 525–37; Jamil Zaki and Kevin N. Ochsner, "The Neuroscience of Empathy: Progress, Pitfalls and Promise," *Nature Neuroscience* 155 (2012): 675–80.

65 **"painful thermal stimulation"** Matthew Botvinick et al., "Viewing Facial Expressions of Pain Engages Cortical Areas Involved in the Direct Experience of Pain," *Neuroimage* 25 (2005): 312.

similar results for children Jean Decety and Kalina J. Michalska, "Neurodevelopmental Changes in the Circuits Underlying Empathy and Sympathy from Childhood to Adulthood," *Developmental Science* 13 (2010): 886–99.

Other research looks at disgust Bruno Wicker et al., "Both of Us Disgusted in *My* Insula: The Common Neural Basis of Seeing and Feeling Disgust," *Neuron* 40 (2003): 655–64.

"2 girls, 1 cup" Michael Agger, "2 Girls 1 Cup 0 Shame," Slate, January 31, 2008, http://www.slate.com/articles/technology/the_browser/2008/01/2_girls_1_cup_0_shame.html.

a clever evolutionary trick For a discussion of simulation theory, see Alvin I. Goldman, *Simulating Minds: The Philosophy, Psychology, and Neuroscience of Mindreading* (New York: Oxford University Press, 2006).

67 **Hickok points out** Hickock, *Myth of Mirror Neurons*.

68 **"not only lowers it"** Adam Smith, *The Theory of Moral Sentiments* (Lawrence, KS: Digireads.com, 2010), 18.

you feel more empathy For example, John T. Lanzetta and Basil G. Englis, "Expectations of Cooperation and Competition and Their Effects on Observers' Vicarious Emotional Responses," *Journal of Personality and Social Psychology* 56 (1989): 543–54. For a review, see Pinker, *Better Angels*.

Or take a study Jean Decety, Stephanie Echols, and Joshua Correll, "The Blame Game: The Effect of Responsibility and Social Stigma on Empathy for Pain," *Journal of Cognitive Neuroscience* 22 (2010): 985–97.

69 **Adam Smith was here** Smith, *Moral Sentiments*, 33.

One European study Grit Hein et al., "Neural Responses to Ingroup and Outgroup Members' Suffering Predict Individual Differences in Costly Helping," *Neuron* 68 (2010): 149–60.

those who repel us Lasana T. Harris and Susan T. Fiske, "Dehumanizing the Lowest of the Low: Neuroimaging Responses to Extreme Out-Groups," *Psychological Science* 17 (2006): 847–53.

70 **one popular metaphor** Thanks to Elliot Sober for pointing this out to me.

71 **"a tale of two systems"** Zaki and Ochsner, "The Neuroscience of Empathy."

"Psychopathic criminals" Christian Keysers and Valeria Gazzola, "Dissociating the Ability and Propensity for Empathy," *Trends in Cognitive Sciences* 18 (2014): 163.

73 **"But if the enthusiasm"** Jean-Jacques Rousseau, *Emile or On Education* (Sioux Falls, SD: NuVision Publications, 2007), 210.

74 **Jonathan Glover tells** Jonathan Glover, *Humanity* (New Haven, CT: Yale University Press, 2012), 379–80.

"For many years" Pinker, *Better Angels*, 575.

75 **disturbed by the screaming** Herbert George Wells, *The Island of Doctor Moreau* (New York: Dover Publications, 1996), 26. Thanks to Christina Starmans for this example.

Batson's own analysis C. Daniel Batson, *Altruism in Humans* (New York: Oxford University Press, 2011).

76 **support the generalization**   For a similar analysis, see Martin L. Hoffman, *Empathy and Moral Development: Implications for Caring and
Justice* (New York: Cambridge University Press, 2001).

78 **well-known scale**   Mark H. Davis, "A Multidimensional Approach to
Individual Differences in Empathy," *JSAS Catalog of Selected Docu-
ments in Psychology* 10 (1980): 85.
    belief in fate   Konika Banerjee and Paul Bloom, "Why Did This Hap-
pen to Me? Religious Believers' and Non-Believers' Teleological Reasoning About Life Events," *Cognition* 133 (2014): 277–303.

81 **Another popular scale**   Simon Baron-Cohen and Sally Wheelwright,
"The Empathy Quotient: An Investigation of Adults with Asperger Syndrome or High Functioning Autism, and Normal Sex Differences," *Journal of Autism and Developmental Disorders* 34 (2004): 163–75.

83 **overall the results are: meh**   Relevant sources here include Bill Under-
wood and Bert Moore, "Perspective-Taking and Altruism," *Psychological
Bulletin* 91 (1982): 143–73; Nancy Eisenberg and Paul A. Miller, "The
Relation of Empathy to Prosocial and Related Behaviors," *Psychological
Bulletin* 101 (1987): 91–119; Steven L. Neuberg et al., "Does Empathy
Lead to Anything More Than Superficial Helping? Comment on Batson
et al. (1997)," *Journal of Personality and Social Psychology* 73 (1997):
510–16; Jesse Prinz, "Is Empathy Necessary for Morality," in *Empathy:
Philosophical and Psychological Perspectives*, eds. Amy Coplan and Peter
Goldie (New York: Oxford University Press, 2011).

84 **"The (Non)Relation between"**   David D. Vachon, Donald R. Lynam,
and Jarrod A. Johnson, "The (Non) Relation Between Empathy and Aggression: Surprising Results from a Meta-Analysis," *Psychological Bulletin* 140 (2014): 16.

Chapter 3: Doing Good

86 **"Empathy-induced altruism"**   C. Daniel Batson et al., "Immorality
from Empathy-Induced Altruism: When Compassion and Justice Conflict," *Journal of Personality and Social Psychology* 68 (1995): 1043 and
1048.

88 **subjects were given $10**   Deborah A. Small and George Loewenstein,

"Helping a Victim or Helping the Victim: Altruism and Identifiability," *Journal of Risk and Uncertainty* 26 (2003): 5–16.

88 **In another study** Ibid.

Other studies compare Tehila Kogut and Ilana Ritov, "The Singularity Effect of Identified Victims in Separate and Joint Evaluations," *Organizational Behavior and Human Decision Processes* 97 (2005): 106–16.

"identifiable victim effect" Thomas C. Schelling, "The Life You Save May Be Your Own," in *Problems in Public Expenditure Analysis*, ed. Samuel B. Chase Jr. (Washington, DC: Brookings Institution, 1968), 128.

90 **"Everybody in America"** Sonia Smith, "Baby Jessica: 25 Years Later," *Texas Monthly*, October 17, 2012, http://www.texasmonthly.com/articles/baby-jessica-25-years-later.

Slovic discusses Paul Slovic, "If I Look at the Mass I Will Never Act: Numbing and Genocide," *Judgment and Decision Making* 2 (2007): 79–95.

91 **"a man of humanity"** Adam Smith, *The Theory of Moral Sentiments* (Lawrence, KS: Digireads.com, 2010), 94.

92 **literature, movies, television** See also Paul Bloom, *Just Babies: The Origins of Good and Evil* (New York: Crown Publishers, 2013).

93 **"Will the world end up"** Walter Isaacson, *Time* essay, December 21, 1992, cited by C. Daniel Batson, *Altruism in Humans* (New York: Oxford University Press, 2011), 198.

"[s]tick-limbed, balloon-bellied" Philip Gourevitch, "Alms Dealers: Can You Provide Humanitarian Aid Without Facilitating Conflicts?" *The New Yorker*, October 11, 2010.

"disaster theory" For example, Enrico Louis Quarantelli, ed., *What Is a Disaster? A Dozen Perspectives on the Question* (London: Routledge, 2005).

96 **consider Peter Singer's example** Peter Singer, *The Most Good You Can Do* (New Haven, CT: Yale University Press, 2016), 6.

99 **"warm glow" givers** Ibid., 5.

consider Western aid Skeptical concerns are raised in several places, including Abhijit Banerjee and Esther Duflo, *Poor Economics: A Radi-*

cal Rethinking of the Way to Fight Global Poverty (New York: PublicAffairs, 2012); William Russell Easterly, *The White Man's Burden: Why the West's Efforts to Aid the Rest Have Done So Much Ill and So Little Good* (New York: Penguin Press, 2006); Ken Stern, *With Charity for All: Why Charities Are Failing and a Better Way to Give* (New York: Anchor Books, 2013); Linda Polman, *The Crisis Caravan: What's Wrong with Humanitarian Aid?* (New York: Macmillan, 2010).

100 **"empathy of foreigners"** Thomas Fuller, "Cambodian Activist's Fall Exposes Broad Deception," *New York Times*, June 14, 2014.

102 **"Effective Altruism"** Kathy Graham, "The Life You Can Save," Happy and Well, May 27, 2013, http://www.happyandwell.com.au/lifesave.

"they don't understand math" Singer, *The Most Good You Can Do*, 87.

As Jennifer Rubenstein put it Jennifer Rubenstein, "Forum: Logic of Effective Altruism," *Boston Review*, July 6, 2015, https://bostonreview.net/forum/logic-effective-altruism/jennifer-rubenstein-response-effective-altruism.

103 **Not everyone is a fan** See the commentators on Peter Singer, "Forum: Logic of Effective Altruism," *Boston Review*, July 6, 2015, https://bostonreview.net/forum/peter-singer-logic-effective-altruism. For further critical remarks on Effective Altruism, see Amia Srinivasan, "Stop the Robot Apocalypse: The New Utilitarians," *London Review of Books*, September 24, 2015.

argument by Scott Alexander Scott Alexander, "Beware Systemic Change," Slate Star Codex, September 22, 2015, http://slatestarcodex.com/2015/09/22/beware-systemic-change.

104 **Larissa MacFarquhar notes** Larissa MacFarquhar, "Forum: Logic of Effective Altruism," https://bostonreview.net/forum/logic-effective-altruism/larissa-macfarquhar-response-effective-altruism.

Paul Brest complains about Paul Brest, "Forum: Logic of Effective Altruism," https://bostonreview.net/forum/logic-effective-altruism/paul-brest-response-effective-altruism.

Catherine Tumber discusses Catherine Tumber, "Forum: Logic of Effective Altruism," https://bostonreview.net/forum/logic-effective-altruism/catherine-tumber-response-effective-altruism.

104 **Singer has less patience** Peter Singer, "Forum: Logic of Effective Altruism, Reply," https://bostonreview.net/forum/logic-effective-altruism/peter-singer-reply-effective-altruism-responses.

106 **One of the most thoughtful** Elaine Scarry, "The Difficulty of Imagining Other People," in *For Love of Country: Debating the Limits of Patriotism*, eds. Martha C. Nussbaum and Joshua Cohen (Boston: Beacon Press, 1996), 102.

107 **philosophers such as Martha Nussbaum** Martha C. Nussbaum, *Upheavals of Thought: The Intelligence of the Emotions* (New York: Cambridge University Press, 2003).
George Eliot argued Steven Pinker, *The Better Angels of Our Nature: Why Violence Has Declined* (New York: Penguin Books, 2011), 589.

109 **"The veil of ignorance"** Scarry, "The Difficulty", 106.
"You just have to want" Louis C.K., cited by Bekka Williams, "Just Want a Shitty Body," in *Louis C.K. and Philosophy*, ed. Mark Ralkowski (Chicago, IL: Open Court).

110 **Simon Baron-Cohen presents** Simon Baron-Cohen, "Forum: Against Empathy," *Boston Review*, August 2014.

112 **"the dismal science"** Tim Harcourt, "No Longer a Dismal Science," *The Spectator*, March 9, 2013, http://www.spectator.co.uk/2013/03/no-longer-a-dismal-science.
"Not a 'gay science'" Ibid.

Interlude: The Politics of Empathy

113 **"Behind every progressive"** George Lakoff, *The Political Mind: A Cognitive Scientist's Guide to Your Brain and Its Politics* (New York: Penguin Books, 2008), 47.

116 **one study asked** Dan Kahan, "Do Mass Political Opinions Cohere: And Do Psychologists 'Generalize Without Evidence' More Often Than Political Scientists?" (New Haven, CT: Cultural Cognition Project at Yale Law School, December 20, 2012), http://www.culturalcognition.net/blog/2012/12/20/do-mass-political-opinions-cohere-and-do-psychologists-gener.html.

116 **political continuum . . . might be universal** Quotes are from John R. Hibbing, Kevin B. Smith, and John R. Alford, "Differences in Negativity Bias Underlie Variations in Political Ideology," *Behavioral and Brain Sciences* 37 (2014): 297–307.

117 **"matters of reproduction"** Ibid., 305.
rough correlation Ibid., 297–307.

118 **"The most important thing"** Peter Baker and Amy Chozick, "Some Conservatives Say Deadly Force Used to Subdue Garner Didn't Fit the Crime," *New York Times*, December 4, 2014.
"To the extent that citizens identify" Clifford P. McCue and J. David Gopoian, "Dispositional Empathy and the Political Gender Gap," *Women and Politics* 21 (2000): 6.

119 **"I like being able to fire people"** Derek Thompson, "The Meaning of Mitt Romney Saying 'I Like Being Able to Fire People,'" *The Atlantic*, January 9, 2012, http://www.theatlantic.com/business/archive/2012/01/the-meaning-of-mitt-romney-saying-i-like-being-able-to-fire-people/251090.
"The very idea" George Lakoff, *Whose Freedom? The Battle Over America's Most Important Idea* (New York: Macmillan, 2006), 193.

120 **worry that these never work** For instance, Thomas Sowell, *A Conflict of Visions: Ideological Origins of Political Struggles* (New York: Basic Books, 2007).
A different analysis Jonathan Haidt, *The Righteous Mind: Why Good People Are Divided by Politics and Religion* (New York: Vintage Books, 2012).
One study, using online Ravi Iyer et al., "Understanding Libertarian Morality: The Psychological Dispositions of Self-Identified Libertarians," *PLOS ONE*, August 21, 2012, http://journals.plos.org/plosone/article?id=10.1371/journal.pone.0042366.

121 **women tend to be** Susan Pinker, *The Sexual Paradox: Men, Women and the Real Gender Gap* (New York: Simon and Schuster: 2009); Simon Baron-Cohen, *The Essential Difference: Male and Female Brains and the Truth About Autism* (New York: Basic Books, 2004).
if males were as empathic McCue and Gopoian, *Women and Politics* 21: 1–20.

122 **the least empathic individuals of all** Iver et al., "Understanding Libertarian Morality."

123 **"I'd probably want a gun, too"** Eliana Johnson, "Obama: If Michelle Lived in Rural Iowa, She'd Want a Gun, Too," *National Review*, April 3, 2013, http://www.nationalreview.com/corner/344619/obama-if-michelle-lived-rural-iowa-shed-want-gun-too-eliana-johnson.

"an American citizen" Eric Bradner, "Former Bush Officials Defend Interrogation Tactics," CNN Politics, December 15, 2014, http://www.cnn.com/2014/12/15/politics/torture-report-reaction-roundup.

125 **in a thoughtful discussion** Thomas Colby, "In Defense of Judicial Empathy," *Minnesota Law Review* 96 (2012): 1944–2015.

Chapter 4: Intimacy

129 **A team of psychologists** David M. Buss, "Sex Differences in Human Mate Preferences: Evolutionary Hypotheses Tested in 37 Cultures," *Behavioral and Brain Sciences* 12.01 (1989): 1–14.

130 **"we are but one"** Adam Smith, *The Theory of Moral Sentiments* (Lawrence, KS: Digireads.com, 2010), 62.

131 **"Where empathy really"** Paul Bloom, "The Baby in the Well: The Case Against Empathy," *The New Yorker* 118 (2013): 118–21.

132 **"Hannah is a psychotherapist"** Simon Baron-Cohen, *The Science of Evil: On Empathy and the Origins of Cruelty* (New York: Basic Books, 2012), 26, 27.

134 **"unmitigated communion"** Vicki S. Helgeson and Heidi L. Fritz, "Unmitigated Agency and Unmitigated Communion: Distinctions from Agency and Communion," *Journal of Research in Personality* 33, (1999): 131–58; Heidi L. Fritz and Vicki S. Helgeson, "Distinctions of Unmitigated Communion from Communion: Self-Neglect and Overinvolvement with Others," *Journal of Personality and Social Psychology* 75 (1998): 121–40; Vicki S. Helgeson and Heidi L. Fritz, "A Theory of Unmitigated Communion," *Personality and Social Psychology Review* 2 (1998): 173–83.

"overly nurturant, intrusive, and self-sacrificing" Helgeson and Fritz, "A theory," 177.

135 **"It's surprising how many"** Barbara Oakley, *Cold-Blooded Kindness:*

Neuroquirks of a Codependent Killer, or Just Give Me a Shot at Loving You, Dear, and Other Reflections on Helping That Hurts (Amherst, NY: Prometheus Books, 2011), 69.

135 **agency and communion** David Bakan, *The Duality of Human Existence: An Essay on Psychology and Religion* (Chicago: Rand McNally, 1966).

stereotypically male . . . stereotypically female See also Janet T. Spence, Robert L. Helmreich, and Carole K. Holahan, "Negative and Positive Components of Psychological Masculinity and Femininity and Their Relationships to Self-Reports of Neurotic and Acting Out Behaviors," *Journal of Personality and Social Psychology* 37 (1979): 1673–82.

136 **if you want to get happy** Elizabeth Dunn and Michael Norton, *Happy Money: The Science of Smarter Spending* (New York: Simon and Schuster, 2013).

138 **Charles Goodman notes** Charles Goodman, *Consequences of Compassion: An Interpretation and Defense of Buddhist Ethics* (New York: Oxford University Press, 2009).

"In contrast to empathy" Tania Singer and Olga M. Klimecki, "Empathy and Compassion," *Current Biology* 24 (2014): R875.

The neurological difference Ibid.

139 **"a warm positive state"** Olga M. Klimecki, Matthieu Ricard, and Tania Singer, "Empathy Versus Compassion: Lessons from 1st and 3rd Person Methods," in *Compassion: Bridging Practice and Science*, eds. Tania Singer and Matthias Bolz (Max Planck Society, 2013), e-book at http://www.compassion-training.org/?lang=en&page=home.

"The empathic sharing" Ibid.

ongoing experiments led by Singer For example, Olga M. Klimecki et al., "Differential Pattern of Functional Brain Plasticity after Compassion and Empathy Training," *Social Cognitive and Affective Neuroscience* 9 (2014): 873–79.

140 **"When experienced chronically** Singer and Klimecki, "Empathy and Compassion."

conclusions of David DeSteno Paul Condon et al., "Meditation Increases Compassionate Responses to Suffering," *Psychological Science*

24 (2013): 2125–27; Daniel Lim, Paul Condon, and David DeSteno, "Mindfulness and Compassion: An Examination of Mechanism and Scalability," *PLOS ONE* 10 (2015): e0118221.

141 **"meditation-based training enables practitioners"** David DeSteno, "The Kindness Cure," *The Atlantic*, July 21, 2015, http://www.the atlantic.com/health/archive/2015/07/mindfulness-meditation-empathy-compassion/398867.

"affective empathy is a precursor" Leonardo Christov-Moore and Marco Iacoboni, "Forum: Against Empathy," *Boston Review*, August 2014, https://bostonreview.net/forum/against-empathy/leonardo-christov-moore-marco-iacoboni-response-against-empathy-iacoboni.

"We can't feel compassion" Lynn E. O'Connor and Jack W. Berry, "Forum: Against Empathy," *Boston Review*, August 2014, https://bos tonreview.net/forum/against-empathy/lynn-e-oconnor-jack-w-berry-response-against-empathy-oconnor.

142 **studies that find a decline** Melanie Neumann et al., "Empathy Decline and Its Reasons: A Systematic Review of Studies with Medical Students and Residents," *Academic Medicine* 86 (2011): 996–1009.

"essential learning objective" Christine Montross, "Forum: Against Empathy," *Boston Review*, August 2014, https://bostonreview.net/forum/against-empathy/christine-montross-response-against-empathy-montross.

"If, while listening" Ibid.

144 **nursing students . . . especially prone** Martin L. Hoffman, *Empathy and Moral Development: Implications for Caring and Justice* (New York: Cambridge University Press, 2001).

145 **"tenderness and aestheticism"** Atul Gawande, "Final Cut. Medical Arrogance and the Decline of the Autopsy," *The New Yorker* 77 (2001): 94–99.

"I cannot advise" Peter Kramer, *Freud: Inventor of the Modern Mind* (New York: HarperCollins, 2006), 26.

146 **"I didn't need him to be"** Leslie Jamison, *The Empathy Exams: Essays* (New York: Macmillan, 2014), 17.

"Still, in most of the interactions" Montross, "Forum: Against Empathy."

147 **"I appreciated the care"** Leslie Jamison, "Forum: Against Empathy," *Boston Review*, August 2014, https://bostonreview.net/forum/against-empathy/leslie-jamison-response-against-empathy-leslie-jamison.

"transformative experiences" Laurie Ann Paul, *Transformative Experience* (New York: Oxford University Press, 2014).

148 **Jackson tells the story of Mary** Frank Jackson, "What Mary Didn't Know," *Journal of Philosophy* 83 (1986): 291–95.

150 **The intricacies here** This discussion is based on Russ Roberts, *How Adam Smith Can Change Your Life: An Unexpected Guide to Human Nature and Happiness* (New York: Portfolio/Penguin, 2014).

151 **"The mind, therefore"** Smith, *Moral Sentiments*, 19.

"small joys" Ibid., 32.

153 **"his brother hummed"** Ibid., 33.

"Nature, it seems" Ibid., 37.

154 **many scholars have argued** For discussion, see C. Daniel Batson, *Altruism in Humans* (New York: Oxford University Press, 2011).

155 **"we put ourselves"** Stephen Darwall, *Honor, History, and Relationship: Essays in Second-Personal Ethics II* (New York: Oxford University Press, 2013), 125–26.

"The father who becomes" Michael Slote, "Reply to Noddings, Darwall, Wren, and Fullinwider," *Theory and Research in Education* 8 (2010): 187–97.

156 **"It should be a sincere"** Heidi Howkins Lockwood, "On Apology Redux," Feminist Philosophers, September 25, 2014, http://feministphilosophers.wordpress.com/2014/09/25/on-apology-redux.

"what makes an apology" Aaron Lazare, *On Apology* (New York: Oxford University Press, 2005), 42.

157 **"A past wrong"** Pamela Hieronymi, "Articulating an Uncompromising Forgiveness," *Philosophy and Phenomenological Research* 62 (2001): 546.

158 **"he is an absolutely"** Norman Finkelstein, ZNet Interview, February 1, 2014, http://normanfinkelstein.com/2014/02/02/an-alienated-finkelstein-discusses-his-writing-being-unemployable-and-noam-chomsky.

159 **Asma begins by describing** Stephen T. Asma, *Against Fairness* (Chicago: University of Chicago Press, 2012), 1.

160 **"The essence of being human"** George Orwell, "Reflections on Gandhi," in *A Collection of Essays* (New York: Harvest, 1970), 176.

Singer argues that For a recent summary of Singer's views, see Peter Singer, *The Most Good You Can Do* (New Haven, CT: Yale University Press, 2016).

161 **As Larissa MacFarquhar** Larissa MacFarquhar, *Strangers Drowning: Grappling with Impossible Idealism, Drastic Choices, and the Overpowering Urge to Help* (New York: Penguin, 2015), 8.

162 **"asks himself"** MacFarquhar, *Strangers Drowning*, 8.

Interlude: Empathy as the Foundation of Morality

166 **Martin Hoffman, for instance** Martin L. Hoffman, *Empathy and Moral Development: Implications for Caring and Justice* (New York: Cambridge University Press, 2001), 4 and 3.

As Michael Ghiselin put it Michael T. Ghiselin, *The Economy of Nature and the Evolution of Sex* (Berkeley: University of California Press, 1976), 247.

167 **"Mr. Lincoln once remarked"** C. Daniel Batson et al., "Where Is the Altruism in the Altruistic Personality?" *Journal of Personality and Social Psychology* 50 (1986): 212–20.

170 **As William James put it** William James, *Psychology: Briefer Course*, vol. 14 (Cambridge, MA: Harvard University Press, 1984), 386.

Frans de Waal has done For example, Frans De Waal, *Primates and Philosophers: How Morality Evolved* (Princeton, NJ; Princeton University Press, 2009).

171 **toddlers do seem to care** For examples of key empirical studies, see Carolyn Zahn-Waxler, Joanne L. Robinson, and Robert N. Emde, "The Development of Empathy in Twins," *Developmental Psychology* 28 (1992): 1038–47, and Carolyn Zahn-Waxler et al., "Development of Concern for Others," *Developmental Psychology* 28 (1992): 126–36.

toddlers will help adults Felix Warneken and Michael Tomasello, "Altruistic Helping in Human Infants and Young Chimpanzees," *Science* 311 (2006): 1301–3; Felix Warneken and Michael Tomasello, "Helping and Cooperation at 14 Months of Age," *Infancy* 11 (2007):

271–94; for review, see Michael Tomasello, *Why We Cooperate* (Cambridge, MA: MIT Press, 2009).

171 **some theorists have argued** Richard Cook et al., "Mirror Neurons: From Origin to Function," *Behavioral and Brain Sciences* 37 (2014): 177–92.

if you stick out your tongue Andrew N. Meltzoff and M. Keith Moore, "Imitation of Facial and Manual Gestures by Human Neonates," *Science* 198 (1977): 75–78.

172 **This is controversial** Cook et al., "Mirror Neurons."

Meltzoff and his colleagues Maria Laura Filippetti et al., "Body Perception in Newborns," *Current Biology* 23 (2013): 2413–16; Maria Laura Filippetti et al., "Newborn Body Perception: Sensitivity to Spatial Congruency," *Infancy* 20 (2015): 455–65; for review and discussion, see Peter J. Marshall and Andrew N. Meltzoff, "Body Maps in the Infant Brain," *Trends in Cognitive Sciences* 19 (2015): 499–505.

Charles Darwin thought so Charles Darwin, "A Biographical Sketch of an Infant," *Mind* 2 (1877): 289.

babies get upset For review, see Hoffman, *Empathy and Moral Development.*

I cited all this Paul Bloom, *Just Babies: The Origins of Good and Evil* (New York: Crown Publishers, 2013).

173 **"retreated to the corner"** G. E. J. Rice, "Aiding Behavior vs. Fear in the Albino Rat," *Psychological Record* 14 (1964): 165–70, cited by Stephanie D. Preston and Frans de Waal, "Empathy: Its Ultimate and Proximate Bases," *Behavioral and Brain Sciences* 25 (2002): 1–71.

174 **Paul Harris has reviewed** Paul Harris, "The Early Emergence of Concern for Others" (unpublished manuscript, Harvard University, n.d.).

"The 15-month-old, Len" Example from Judy Dunn and Carol Kendrick, *Siblings: Love, Envy, and Understanding* (Cambridge, MA: Harvard University Press, 1982), 115.

175 **consider a classic study** Dale F. Hay, Alison Nash, and Jan Pedersen, "Responses of Six-Month-Olds to the Distress of Their Peers," *Child Development* (1981): 1071–75.

an observation about chimpanzees Frans B. M. De Waal and Filippo

Aureli, "Consolation, Reconciliation, and a Possible Cognitive Difference Between Macaques and Chimpanzees," *Reaching into Thought: The Minds of the Great Apes* (1996): 80–110.

175 **Paul Harris points out** Harris, "Early Emergence."

Chapter 5: Violence and Cruelty

177 **In April of 1945** Steve Friess, "A Liberator but Never Free," *The New Republic*, May 17, 2015, http://www.newrepublic.com/article/121779/liberator-never-free.

179 **Some see certain violent actions** Michael R. Gottfredson and Travis Hirschi, *A General Theory of Crime* (Stanford, CA: Stanford University Press, 1990).

alcohol and other drugs Roy F. Baumeister, *Evil: Inside Human Violence and Cruelty* (New York: Macmillan, 1999).

a kind of cancer Adrian Raine, *The Anatomy of Violence: The Biological Roots of Crime* (New York: Vintage Books, 2013).

violence is an essential part Paul Bloom, "Natural-Born Killers," *New York Times Sunday Book Review*, June 21, 2013.

180 **"the myth of pure evil"** Baumeister, *Evil*, 17.

181 **Smith also notes** David Livingstone Smith, *Less Than Human: Why We Demean, Enslave, and Exterminate Others* (New York: Macmillan, 2011).

"the moralization gap" Steven Pinker, *The Better Angels of Our Nature: Why Violence Has Declined* (New York: Penguin Books, 2011).

The most extreme example Baumeister, *Evil*, 6.

In one study, Baumeister Roy F. Baumeister, Arlene Stillwell, and Sara R. Wotman, "Victim and Perpetrator Accounts of Interpersonal Conflict: Autobiographical Narratives About Anger," *Journal of Personality and Social Psychology* 59 (1990): 994–1005.

183 **"If we as social scientists"** Roy F. Baumeister, "Human Evil: The Myth of Pure Evil and the True Causes of Violence," in *The Social Psychology of Morality: Exploring the Causes of Good and Evil*, eds. Mario Mikulincer and Philip. R. Shaver (Washington, DC: American Psychological Association, 2012).

184 **"The world has far too much"** Pinker, *Better Angels*, 622.

184 **"It's always the good men"** Baumeister, *Evil*, 169.

Tage Rai, summarizing Tage Rai, "How Could They?" *Aeon Magazine*, June 18, 2015, http://aeon.co/magazine/philosophy/people-do-violence-because-their-moral-codes-demand-it.

185 **I read a story** Caroline Mortimer, "Man Let Daughter Drown Rather Than Have Strange Men Touch Her, Dubai Police Claim," *The Independent*, August 10, 2015, http://www.independent.co.uk/news/world/middle-east/man-lets-daughter-drown-rather-than-let-strange-men-touch-her-10448008.html.

188 **"I did not shoot"** Cited by Jonathan Glover, *Humanity* (New Haven, CT: Yale University Press, 2012), 115.

"Consider Israeli Prime Minister" Simon Baron-Cohen, "Forum: Against Empathy," *Boston Review*, August 2014, https://bostonreview.net/forum/against-empathy/simon-baron-cohen-response-against-empathy-baron-cohen.

191 **In World War II** Thanks to Max Bloom for this example.

"When we see one man" Adam Smith, *The Theory of Moral Sentiments* (Lawrence, KS: Digireads.com, 2010), 98–99.

192 **Ann Coulter's recent book** Ann Coulter, *Adios, America: The Left's Plan to Turn Our Country into a Third World Hellhole* (Washington, DC: Regnery Publishing, 2015).

193 **a suggestive pair of studies** Anneke E. K. Buffone and Michael J. Poulin, "Empathy, Target Distress, and Neurohormone Genes Interact to Predict Aggression for Others—Even Without Provocation," *Personality and Social Psychology Bulletin* 40 (2014): 1406–22.

195 **We tell our subjects stories** Michael N. Stagnaro and Paul Bloom, "The Paradoxical Effects of Empathy on the Willingness to Punish" (unpublished manuscript, Yale University, 2016).

196 **concern that many Nazis had** Arnold Arluke, *Regarding Animals* (Philadelphia: Temple University Press, 1996), 152.

197 **Jennifer Skeem and her colleagues** Jennifer L. Skeem et al., "Psychopathic Personality: Bridging the Gap Between Scientific Evidence and Public Policy," *Psychological Science in the Public Interest* 12 (2011): 95–162.

197 **The traits that comprise** The table is from ibid.

199 **Some have argued** Ibid.

"deficient empathy, disdain" Ibid.

200 **as Jesse Prinz points out** Jesse Prinz, "Is Empathy Necessary for Morality," in *Empathy: Philosophical and Psychological Perspectives*, eds. Amy Coplan and Peter Goldie (New York: Oxford University Press, 2011).

"Vexation, spite" Hervey M. Cleckley, *The Mask of Sanity: An Attempt to Clarify Some Issues About the So-Called Psychopathic Personality* (Augusta, GA: Emily S. Cleckley, 1988), cited by Prinz, "Is Empathy Necessary."

A different concern is raised Skeem et al., "Psychopathic Personality."

201 **a meta-analysis summarized** David D. Vachon, Donald R. Lynam, and Jarrod A. Johnson, "The (Non) Relation Between Empathy and Aggression: Surprising Results from a Meta-Analysis," *Psychological Bulletin* 140 (2014): 751–73.

People with Asperger's syndrome Ruth C. M. Philip et al., "A Systematic Review and Meta-Analysis of the fMRI Investigation of Autism Spectrum Disorders," *Neuroscience and Biobehavioral Reviews* 36 (2012): 901–42. See also Simon Baron-Cohen, *The Science of Evil: On Empathy and the Origins of Cruelty* (New York: Basic Books, 2012).

Baron-Cohen points out Baron-Cohen, *Science of Evil*.

202 **Some of the most interesting** Smith, *Less Than Human*.

the missionary Morgan Godwin Ibid., 115.

203 **"Humankind ceases at the border of the tribe"** Jacques-Philippe Leyens et al., "The Emotional Side of Prejudice: The Attribution of Secondary Emotions to Ingroups and Outgroups," *Personality and Social Psychology Review* 4 (2000): 186–97.

In laboratory studies Leyens et al., "Emotional Side of Prejudice." See also Nick Haslam, "Dehumanization: An Integrative Review," *Personality and Social Psychology Review* 10 (2006): 252–64.

Feminist scholars Andrea Dworkin, *Pornography: Men Possessing Women* (New York: Putnam Press, 1981); Catharine A MacKinnon, *Only Words* (Cambridge, MA: Harvard University Press, 1993); Martha C. Nussbaum, "Objectification," *Philosophy and Public Affairs* 24 (1995): 249–91. For review, see Evangelia Papadaki, "Sexual Objectification: From Kant to Contemporary Feminism," *Contemporary Political Theory* 6 (2007): 330–48.

203 **Martha Nussbaum suggests** Nussbaum, "Objectification," 257.

dehumanization, not objectification For a brief discussion of this idea (I hope to write more in the future), see Paul Bloom, "The Ways of Lust," *New York Times*, December 1, 2013.

204 **"Come on dogs"** Smith, *Less Than Human*, 11.

205 **Kate Manne makes a similar argument** Kate Manne, "In Ferguson and Beyond, Punishing Humanity," *New York Times*, October 12, 2014.

"acknowledge their victims'" Kwame Anthony Appiah, *Experiments in Ethics* (Cambridge, MA: Harvard University Press, 2008), 144.

206 **a large body of experimental research** Kurt Gray et al., "More Than a Body: Mind Perception and the Nature of Objectification," *Journal of Personality and Social Psychology* 101 (2011): 1207–20.

"Treating other people" Baron-Cohen, *Science of Evil*, 8.

Smith points out David Livingstone Smith, "Paradoxes of Dehumanization," *Social Theory and Practice* 42 (2016): 416–43.

207 **"The SS escort"** Primo Levi, *The Drowned and the Saved* (London: Abacus, 1988), 70–71.

A couple is lying in bed Nussbaum, "Objectification."

208 **Owen Flanagan once described** Owen Flanagan, *The Geography of Morals: Varieties of Possibility* (New York: Oxford University Press, 2017), 158.

209 **angry subjects were more punitive** Jennifer S. Lerner, Julie H. Goldberg, and Philip E. Tetlock, "Sober Second Thought: The Effects of Accountability, Anger, and Authoritarianism on Attributions of Responsibility," *Personality and Social Psychology Bulletin* 24 (1998): 563–74.

210 **Flanagan sadly concedes this** Flanagan, *The Geography of Morals*.

"Righteous rage is a cornerstone" Jesse Prinz, "Forum: Against Empathy," *Boston Review*, August 2014, https://bostonreview.net/forum/against-empathy/jesse-prinz-response-against-empathy-prinz.

Chapter 6: Age of Reason

213 **Age of Reason** Some of this chapter is a substantially modified version of Paul Bloom, "The War on Reason," *The Atlantic*, March 2014,

http://www.theatlantic.com/magazine/archive/2014/03/the-war-on-reason/357561.

213 **the Third Pounder** The story is told by Elizabeth Green, "Why Do Americans Stink at Math," *New York Times Magazine, July 23, 2014.*

214 *Thinking, Fast and Slow* Daniel Kahneman, *Thinking, Fast and Slow* (New York: Macmillan, 2011).

I recently wrote Paul Bloom, "Imagining the Lives of Others," *New York Times,* June 6, 2015.

218 **"a biochemical puppet"** Sam Harris, *Free Will* (New York: Simon and Schuster, 2012), 47.

David Eagleman makes this argument David Eagleman, *Incognito: The Secret Lives of the Brain* (New York: Pantheon, 2011).

219 **"It is not clear"** Ibid., 46.

220 **One scholar, for instance** Cited in Paul Bloom, "My Brain Made Me Do It," *Journal of Cognition and Culture* 6 (2006): 212. See also Joshua Greene and Jonathan Cohen, "For the Law, Neuroscience Changes Nothing and Everything," *Philosophical Transactions of the Royal Society of London B* 359 (2004): 1775–85.

"My brain made me do it" Michael S. Gazzaniga, *The Ethical Brain: The Science of Our Moral Dilemmas* (New York: Dana Press, 2005).

221 **countless demonstrations** For a good review of these experiments and others, see Adam Alter, *Drunk Tank Pink: And Other Unexpected Forces That Shape How We Think, Feel, and Behave* (New York: Penguin Books, 2013).

222 **Dick Finder** Example from John M. Doris, *Talking to Our Selves: Reflection, Ignorance, and Agency* (Oxford: Oxford University Press, 2015).

223 **Jonathan Haidt captures** Jonathan Haidt, "The Emotional Dog and Its Rational Tail: A Social Intuitionist Approach to Moral Judgment," *Psychological Review* 108 (2001): 814–34.

The issue in "repligate" For discussion, see Paul Bloom, "Psychology's Replication Crisis Has a Silver Lining," *The Atlantic,* February 19, 2016, http://www.theatlantic.com/science/archive/2016/02/psychology-studies-replicate/468537.

224 **eventually published this failure** Brian D. Earp et al., "Out, Damned

Spot: Can the 'Macbeth Effect' Be Replicated?" *Basic and Applied Social Psychology* 36 (2014): 91–98.

224 **Your impression of a résumé** Joshua M. Ackerman, Christopher C. Nocera, and John A. Bargh, "Incidental Haptic Sensations Influence Social Judgments and Decisions," *Science* 328 (2010): 1712–15.

225 **Your assessment of gay people** Yoel Inbar, David A. Pizarro, and Paul Bloom, "Disgusting Smells Cause Decreased Liking of Gay Men," *Emotion* 12 (2012): 23–27.

people eat less Brian Wansink, *Mindless Eating: Why We Eat More Than We Think* (New York: Bantam Books, 2007).

226 **psychologists put baseball cards** Ian Ayres, Mahzarin R. Banaji, and Christine Jolls, "Race Effects on eBay," *Rand Journal of Economics* 46 (2015): 891–917.

other well-known demonstrations For review, see Kahneman, *Thinking, Fast and Slow.*

228 **"mind bugs"** Mahzarin R. Banaji and Anthony G. Greenwald, *Blind Spot: Hidden Biases of Good People* (New York: Delacorte Press, 2013).

229 **John Macnamara pointed out** John Theodore Macnamara, *A Border Dispute: The Place of Logic in Psychology* (Cambridge, MA: MIT Press, 1986).

231 **"are *obsessed* with intelligence"** Steven Pinker, *The Blank Slate: The Modern Denial of Human Nature* (Penguin Books, 2003), 149.

As David Brooks writes David Brooks, *The Social Animal: The Hidden Sources of Love, Character, and Achievement* (New York: Random House, 2012), xi.

Malcolm Gladwell . . . argues Malcolm Gladwell, *Outliers* (Boston: Little, Brown, 2008), 76.

232 **IQ is critically important** For a good review of the state of the art here, see David Z. Hambrick and Christopher Chabris, "Yes, IQ Really Matters," Slate, April 14, 2014, http://www.slate.com/articles/health_and_science/science/2014/04/what_do_sat_and_iq_tests_measure_general_intelligence_predicts_school_and.html.

233 **professional moral philosophers** Eric Schwitzgebel and Joshua Rust, "The Moral Behavior of Ethics Professors: Relationships Among Self-

Reported Behavior, Expressed Normative Attitude, and Directly Observed Behavior," *Philosophical Psychology* 27 (2014): 293–327.

234 **Walter Mischel investigated**   For a review, see Walter Mischel, *The Marshmallow Test: Mastering Self-Control* (Boston: Little, Brown, 2014).

studies of exceptional altruists   Abigail A. Marsh et al., "Neural and Cognitive Characteristics of Extraordinary Altruists," *Proceedings of the National Academy of Sciences* 111 (2014): 15036–41.

Steven Pinker has argued   Steven Pinker, *The Better Angels of Our Nature: Why Violence Has Declined* (New York: Penguin Books, 2011).

235 **Smith discusses the qualities**   Adam Smith, *The Theory of Moral Sentiments* (Lawrence, KS: Digireads.com, 2010), 130.

studies run by Geoffrey Cohen   Geoffrey L. Cohen, "Party Over Policy: The Dominating Impact of Group Influence on Political Beliefs," *Journal of Personality and Social Psychology* 85 (2003): 808–22.

236 **Other studies have found**   Philip M. Fernbach et al., "Political Extremism Is Supported by an Illusion of Understanding," *Psychological Science* 24 (2013): 939–46.

238 **"they don't understand math"**   Peter Singer, *The Most Good You Can Do* (New Haven, CT: Yale University Press, 2016), 87.

"Numbers turned me into an altruist"   Ibid., 88.

239 **People are not at a loss**   Paul Bloom, *Just Babies: The Origins of Good and Evil* (New York: Crown Publishers, 2013).

As scholars like Steven Pinker   Pinker, *Better Angels*; Peter Singer, *The Expanding Circle* (Oxford: Clarendon Press, 1981); Robert Wright, *Nonzero: The Logic of Human Destiny* (New York: Vintage Books, 2001).

240 **"The Old Testament tells us"**   Pinker, *Better Angels*, 591.

"It is not the soft power"   Smith, *Moral Sentiments*, 95.

Index

arguments against empathy
(*continued*)
   morality without empathy, 22–26
   use of terms, 16–17, 35–36,
     39–41
Aristotle, 213, 216
Asma, Stephen, 159, 160–61
Asperger's syndrome, 201
Assad, Bashar al-, 193
assessment of empathy, 77–83
Atlantic, The, 11
authority, and conservatives, 119, 120
autism, 20, 81, 82, 201
autonomy, 150, 203

babies
   empathy in, 171–76
   morality in, 6, 165, 171
Bakan, David, 135
Baldwin, Jason, 25, 27
Baron-Cohen, Simon, 201, 206
   bad people and empathy, 20–21,
     201
   decision making and empathy,
     110–11, 188–89, 190, 191
   empathizer scale, 81–82, 121,
     195
   high empathy in personal
     relationships, 132–33, 136
Batkid (Miles Scott), 96–97
Batman (character), 180
Batson, C. Daniel, 25, 58–59
   empathy-altruism hypothesis,
     75–76, 83, 85–87, 168

   Sheri Summers experiment, 25,
     86–87
Baumeister, Roy, 180, 181–82, 183
Bazelon, Emily, 20
beggars, 74, 100, 105
Bentham, Jeremy, 29
Berry, Jack W., 141
Biafra famine, 93
biases, 9, 48–49, 50, 89–101, 109
Bin Laden, Osama, 186
Bleak House (Dickens), 48–49, 160,
   161
"Blood is thicker than water," 7–8,
   159
Boston Red Sox, 236
Boston Review, 11, 12, 103
boxing, and violence, 187
brain. *See* neuroscience
Brazelton, T. Berry, 18–19
Brest, Paul, 104
Brooks, David, 231–32
Brotherhood of Evil Mutants
   (fictional), 180
Brothers Karamazov, The
   (Dostoyevsky), 178
Buddha (Buddhism), 137–38,
   149–50, 161, 208–9
Buffone, Anneke, 193–95
bullies (bullying), 20, 30–31, 37
"burnout," 137
Bush, George, 235

calmness, 146
Cambodian orphanages, 100

Mother Teresa of Calcutta, 89
Myth of Mirror Neurons, The
    (Hickok), 64, 67

names (naming), 222
national disasters, and election years,
    94
natural selection, 168–70
Nazi Doctors, The (Lifton), 16
Nazis, 5, 16, 74, 110–11, 124,
    177–78, 181, 191, 196, 202,
    206–7
Netanyahu, Benjamin, 188–89, 190
neuroscience, 47, 59–73
    of compassion, 138–39
    difference between feeling and
        understanding, 70–73
    of empathic experiences, 62–68
    empathic reactions and
        prior bias, preference, and
        judgment, 68–70, 90
    localization problem, 59–61
    other people's pain, 62–68, 73–75
    of reason, 216–21
Newtown school shooting, 1–2,
    31–33, 90
New Yorker, The, 11–12
New York Times, 11, 100, 214
Nussbaum, Martha, 10, 107, 203

Oakley, Barbara, 135
Obama, Barack, 2, 4, 18, 19, 118,
    119, 122–23, 235
Obama, Michelle, 123

objectification, 178–79, 203–4, 206
objectivity, 86, 146
Ochsner, Kevin, 71–72
O'Connor, Lynn E., 141
Oliver Twist (Dickens), 92
Omnivore's Dilemma, The (Pollan),
    50
On Apology (Lazare), 156–57
origins of empathy, 171–76
orphanages, in Cambodia, 100
Orwell, George, 37–38, 159–60, 188
oxytocin, 195

pain
    babies and empathy, 172–74
    neuroscience of, 62–68, 73–75
    role in empathy, 17, 21, 33–36,
        62–68, 155–56
parenting, 97, 130–31, 154–55
Parkinson's disease, 219
parochialism, 9, 36
"pathological altruism," 135
Patton, George S., 178
Paul, Laurie, 147–48
Paul, Ron, 118
Personal Concern scale, 80–81
personal distress, 25
Personal Distress scale, 79–81
Perspective Taking scale, 78–81
physicalism, 148
physician-patient relationship,
    143–45, 146–47
Pinker, Steven, 10, 18–19, 74–75,
    239–40